PRAISE FOR
EATING FOR RECOVERY:

"As a physician, I have found that alcoholism is always accompanied by nutritional imbalances. Following an excellent nutritional program makes recovery from this problem much easier and more effective. With its recipes, menus, and nutritional advice, this wonderful book by Molly Siple is a very helpful resource for anyone recovering from this condition."

—SUSAN LARK, MD, AUTHOR OF
DR. SUSAN LARK'S HORMONE REVOLUTION

"This book is an invaluable, science-based guide providing all the tools for incorporating good nutrition in the recovery process."

—BARRY S. SOLOF, MD, FASAM,
REGIONAL CHIEF, ADDICTION MEDICINE,
SOUTHERN CALIFORNIA PERMANENTE MEDICAL GROUP

"Sensible, practical, life-changing! A must-have for every person in recovery—and their family members too."

—KATHERINE KETCHAM, COAUTHOR
BEYOND THE INFLUENCE: UNDERSTANDING AND DEFEATING ALCOHOLISM AND EATING RIGHT TO STAY SOBER

EATING FOR RECOVERY

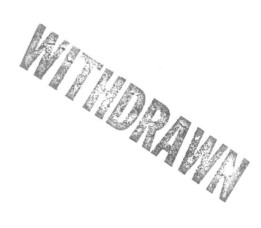

ABOUT THE AUTHOR

Molly Siple, MS, RD, a registered dietitian with a scientific background in nutrition, is an expert in the field after more than twenty years of experience in food and health. Siple's culinary interests began with the launch of her highly successful catering business in New York City. She went on to teach nutrition at the prestigious Southern California Cordon Bleu School of Culinary Arts. She has authored/coauthored more than ten books, including *Healing Foods for Dummies* and *Recipes for Change,* which was a nominee for the International Association of Culinary Professionals' Julia Child Cookbook Awards. Currently on the advisory board of *Natural Health* magazine, Siple has appeared as a nutrition spokesperson on ABCTV–7 in Los Angeles and the *Today Show.* She lives in Los Angeles. Her Web site is eatingforrecovery.com.

EATING FOR RECOVERY

*The Essential Nutrition Plan
to Reverse the Physical Damage
of Alcoholism*

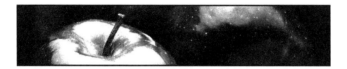

MOLLY SIPLE, MS, RD

Da Capo
LIFE
LONG

A Member of the Perseus Books Group

Many of the designations used by manufacturers and sellers to distinguish their products are claimed as trademarks. Where those designations appear in this book and Da Capo Press was aware of a trademark claim, the designations have been printed in initial capital letters.

Designed by Lisa Kreinbrink
Set in 12-point ACaslon by the Perseus Books Group

Library of Congress Cataloging-in-Publication Data

Siple, Molly.
    Eating for recovery : the essential nutrition plan to reverse the physical damage of alcoholism / Molly Siple.—1st ed.
        p.   cm.
    Includes bibliographical references and index.
    ISBN 978-1-60094-044-6 (alk. paper)
    1. Alcoholism—Diet therapy.   2. Alcoholism—Nutritional aspects.   I. Title.
RC565.S535   2008
616.86'10654—dc22

                                                                              2008017425

First Da Capo Press edition 2008

Published by Da Capo Press
A Member of the Perseus Books Group
www.dacapopress.com

Da Capo Press books are available at special discounts for bulk purchases in the United States by corporations, institutions, and other organizations. For more information, please contact the Special Markets Department at the Perseus Books Group, 2300 Chestnut Street, Suite 200, Philadelphia, PA 19103, or call (800) 810-4145, extension 5000, or e-mail special.markets@perseusbooks.com.

1 2 3 4 5 6 7 8 9

To our friend Peter.

CONTENTS

1 GOOD NUTRITION

An Essential Part of Your Recovery Process

NOT LONG AGO, my friend and I waved good-bye to her husband as we left to drive to a school reunion. Six hours later, we were standing by his lifeless body, laid out on a bed in a hospital emergency room. He had died of a massive heart attack just a year and a half after entering an alcohol recovery program and quitting drinking.

I knew that this man had so far been successful in his recovery program—staying away from his typical binge drinking and regularly attending alcoholism support meetings. In our last conversation together that afternoon he had said how good he felt about himself and where he found himself in life—a happy man. But I also knew that he began his days by skipping breakfast, grabbing a scant lunch at most, and then loading up on a well-balanced dinner, finished off with a rich dessert, while drinking coffee from morning to night. He had also picked up his old habit of smoking cigarettes.

In the days and weeks that followed this sorrowful event, I kept wishing that, as a nutritionist, I had had the chance to prevent my friend's untimely death. I could understand how someone focusing on staying abstinent could overlook the importance of diet in his recovery process. I also realized how much I wanted to help others fill in that missing part so that at least they could avoid health problems linked to their drinking days. I began to explore the association between surviving alcoholism and diet. I was well aware of the powerful effect food has on all our body systems and now I wanted to know more about how alcohol played into this. I also wanted to develop a list of specific foods that, eaten regularly, could help reverse damage from alcohol and increase someone's odds for living a long and healthy life. The result of my investigations, as I read the medical literature, became this book. The nutrition program it offers can ease your process of recovery as your health improves and may even help you stay sober.

One reason people who drink too much develop health problems is poor nutrition, adding to the damage that alcohol inflicts. This fact was summed up in an editorial appearing in a 1989 issue of the *New England Journal of Medicine* that stated that excessive alcohol consumption is probably responsible for most of the medical disorders associated with abusing drink, and that malnutrition increases these adverse effects.

Improving eating habits deserves to be an essential part of any recovery regimen. You need to look no further than the following chapters for guidance on how to do this. You'll find practical tips for recovery eating, targeted lists of recovery foods, and over 130 recipes. Use this book for reference and as a cookbook. It's meant to be a powerful tool you can turn to for help fostering your recovery, restoring your health, and ensuring your well-being for years to come. Stopping drinking is an enormous achievement. You deserve a huge amount of credit for having the determination and faith it takes to remain abstinent. Now why not include good nutrition as well in your recovery process? Decide to do this and this book is here to support you. By taking action, you'll reap huge rewards. You can look forward to some great eating and to feeling better than you have for years. Wait until you sample the recommended dishes, like sweet red peppers sautéed in olive oil, oranges scented with cinnamon, spicy fish tacos, and slow-cooked chicken topped with corn custard. Recipes for these and many other delights are incorporated into the eating-for-recovery nutrition plan.

The nutrition-recovery program targets seven goals for healthy eating, ranging from basics, such as making sure to eat breakfast, to cooking with organic ingredients. Aiming for these goals sets you on the path to having more unprocessed and unrefined, natural ingredients in your meals while helping you to cut back on junk food and caffeine. The program is easy to start and you'll be asked to make only small, gradual changes to achieve realistic and quickly attainable results, such as restoring a good appetite, improving your digestion, and beginning to steady your blood sugar.

This program is about moving you in the right direction toward better eating, and it can be taken at your own speed. I'm giving you twenty-one days' worth of menus to help you get started. As you sample and experiment with these, you'll be making the necessary changes in your diet quite naturally. Give yourself three weeks of eating for recovery and you'll be on your way to having new and healthier tastes in food. Give yourself three months and you'll also be feeling noticeably better. While recovery eating brings into your life the fascinating world of food and cooking as well as many new pleasures, this program is especially designed to improve your health. The recovery foods included in the meals and recipes supply the many nutrients that may have become deficient because of heavy drinking.

Recovery Eating for Long-term Health

This nutritional program also helps prevent and reverse the development of a wide range of ailments linked to alcoholism, from digestive problems and fatty liver to degenerative diseases such as heart disease, osteoporosis, and even cancer. (Chapter 2 gives you an overview of these.)

The eating recommendations are backed up by an abundance of studies that demonstrate the ability of good nutrition to ward off and remedy these conditions. Here are just a few of them:

▸ In research focusing on coronary heart disease, authors of a study published in 2002 in the *Journal of the American Medical Association* assessed the findings of 147 investigations involving diet. They identified three eating strategies proven effective for preventing heart disease: (1) substituting saturated fats and trans fats with healthier fats; (2) increasing intake of omega-3 fatty acids (which are found in fish and some plants); and (3) consuming a diet high in vegetables, nuts, and whole grains and low in refined-grain products.

▸ Whole grains were given a thumbs-up for lowering the risk of diabetes, in a Danish study published in 2006 in the *American Journal of Clinical Nutrition*. Among the more than nine hundred men and women in the study, those who reported consuming the most whole grains had better-controlled blood sugar.

▸ A diet providing a wide range of vitamins and minerals, in addition to calcium, helps prevent osteoporosis. This is the conclusion of a paper written by Alan R. Gaby, MD, and Jonathan V. Wright, MD, published in 1988. The authors warn against the typical American diet, high in refined foods and sugar. Whole foods and a variety of produce can supply the additional nutrients that maintaining healthy bone requires. These include vitamins B_6, C, D, and K; and copper, folic acid, magnesium, manganese, silicon, and strontium. Drinking alcohol tends to promote deficiencies of several of these nutrients.

▸ A predominantly plant-based diet, high in a variety of produce, legumes, and minimally processed grains, can play a role in preventing cancer. In 1997, the American Institute for Cancer Research and the World Cancer Research Fund published a comprehensive report, based on an analysis of over 4,500 research studies, which came to this conclusion. Protection against cancer was strongest for diets high in vegetables and fruit. These foods particularly lowered the risk of cancers of the upper digestive tract and, to some extent, the liver, all cancers associated with alcoholism.

You have the opportunity to benefit greatly from all this research, simply by following the recovery eating plan in this book.

Starting Abstinence with Support from Recovery Foods

Besides reducing the risk of various diseases, the recommended foods reduce symptoms associated with the early stages of abstinence. Starting to have regular meals can help control unstable blood sugar levels, an issue for the great majority of alcoholics and a condition that can continue even after drinking has ceased. Certain foods improve digestion and enhance the absorption of nutrients. In addition, for some people, avoiding foods they are sensitive to can lower the risk of relapse, if they are in a habit of turning to alcohol to ease the symptoms of food allergy. (You can find out more about the relationship between food allergy and alcoholism in chapter 4.)

In some cases, what people choose to eat can help them stay away from alcohol. Eating better may improve health to such an extent that life itself becomes more manageable, removing stress that can increase the chance that a person may reach for a drink. Good nutrition can increase energy and mental clarity and help steady mood, making it easier to get through the day. The worse your former diet, the greater the chance you'll soon be feeling better as you switch to recovery foods. Of course, each individual's path of recovery is unique, with its own challenges and roadblocks. Give food a chance to help you heal. You might be surprised by the support it can give you.

Enhancing Detox with Special Ingredients

Many of the foods recommended for recovery eating were selected because they contain substances that play a role in the detoxification processes that go into action automatically within your body as you begin to abstain from alcohol. Once drinking has stopped, some alcohol and by-products of alcohol metabolism still remain in the system and need to be eliminated. The liver is the prime organ involved in detoxification. All sorts of foods support this vitally important liver function: putting together meals that feature vegetables, fruits, grains, and legumes, rather than meats, is called for,

Withdrawal Requires Special Care

In the first hours and days after stopping drinking, withdrawal from alcohol triggers symptoms that can vary greatly. These are usually in relation to how long a person has been an alcoholic and the degree of his or her dependence. They will typically experience a mild to severe hangover that will last several days. Symptoms can include stomach upset, headache, and anxiety. Poor appetite and a delicate stomach are common, as well as dehydration. At this time, having several small meals and grazing is better tolerated rather than eating one large meal. Easy-to-digest soups and vegetarian dishes are also appropriate, with only small amounts of chicken or fish added if desired. Water, fruit and vegetables juices, broth, and herbal teas are the best beverage choices. Chapters 5 and 6 give you lots of options to prepare meals made up of these foods. You'll see this symbol 🦢 next to recipes that are especially easy to digest and mildly flavored, making them helpful during withdrawal.

In addition, for severe withdrawal and its effect on emotions, tranquilizers may be needed. Heavy drinkers, consuming eight to ten drinks a day, may even require treatment in a hospital or inpatient facility to help them through withdrawal. Even if you've adequately tolerated your first days of abstaining, still consider making an appointment with a physician to have a checkup and some blood work to assess your current status of health, information that can help you set a course of action for healing.

as well as cutting back on sugar and fat. This way of eating lightens the burden on the liver, saving its metabolic resources for cleansing. You'll find a variety of dishes in the following chapters that can help you shift your diet in this important direction.

Taking a Look at What You've Been Eating

Think over what you ate in your drinking days. How well did you feed yourself? Maybe you had your share of fruits and vegetables, fish, whole grains, legumes, and so forth. But, more than likely, your diet followed the eating habits of the typical heavy drinker. A large study conducted by the National Institute on Alcohol Abuse and Alcoholism, published in 2006, concluded that people who drink the most, even infrequently, have the poorest eating habits. Researchers measured diet quality using the U.S. Department of Agriculture's Healthy Eating Index. This factors in compliance with the USDA's food guide pyramid, which gives recommendations for number of servings of vegetables, fruits, grains, dairy products, and protein sources such as meats, poultry, fish, eggs, beans, and nuts. Consumption of fat, saturated fat, sodium, cholesterol, and variety of foods was also taken into account. The results of this study showed that the diets of participants were short on foods like fruits and vegetables and long on fat, sodium, and cholesterol. The typical heavy drinker's diet also lacked variety. While this study did not focus specifically on alcoholics, the results did show that as drinking increased, the healthfulness of the diet declined.

There's also lots of anecdotal evidence of how eating habits suffer when drinking pervades a person's lifestyle. Some alcoholics skip meals and drink instead. It's estimated that among Americans who drink too much, one-fifth to one-half of total daily intake of calories is contributed by alcohol. Meals become haphazard. A person holed up at home and drinking may routinely order in pizza when hunger pangs hit and never sit down to a balanced meal. Expense account meals in upscale restaurants are not necessarily much better if a drinker, ordering from a steak and potatoes menu, never touches the vegetables. Some alcoholics, suffering from low self-esteem, have difficulty taking care of themselves. For them, a home-cooked meal is rare and fast foods and snacking become the rule. You probably have your own story to add to these examples.

Whatever your past eating history, here is a chance to start fresh. Beginning with the menus and recipes in this book, starting now, you can shape up your diet and eat for recovery. Try out your cooking skills and explore new foods. Browse through those whole foods emporiums and ethnic food shops, if you haven't done so already. You have much to look forward to discovering. Food will likely soon taste better, as you eat higher-quality foods and your health improves. Cooking may even become your new hobby. Spending a few hours in the kitchen preparing some delectable creation can certainly ease stress and cooking also gives you a way of socializing with others, sharing food rather than getting together over drinks. Letting others cook with you also has benefits, offering family members and friends a healthy way to support you on your path to recovery. In this case, too many cooks won't spoil the broth!

If you've not been feeding your body properly, it's never too late to make amends. The following chapters are full of eating advice and recipes to help you do this. Here's what you'll find in each chapter.

Chapter 2 gives you plenty of reasons to give yourself recovery foods to nourish your body back to health. It offers an overview of the many ailments associated with drinking too much and tells you which recovery recipes are good for which condition. Chapter 2 is also meant to be a wake-up call for family members and friends of alcoholics who may not realize the physical harm that alcohol can inflict. If intervention is being considered, chapter 2 underscores the need to take action now.

Chapter 3 introduces you to the recovery way of eating, pointing you in the direction of fresh, unprocessed, colorful, and organic foods. You'll learn about the right mix of protein, fat, and carbohydrate to have in your meals. This chapter also tells you which vitamins and minerals alcohol abuse can deplete and lists the foods that can replenish these. You'll also find food remedies for various alcohol-related conditions, such as problems with blood sugar, digestion, detoxification, and chronic inflammation.

Next, chapter 4 presents the nutrition program for recovery and introduces and explains the seven goals of recovery eating. There are also handy shopping lists to make stocking up on recovery foods easy. Chapter 5 then shows you how to turn these foods into meals, with twenty-one days' worth of menus based on the recommended ingredients. You'll also find suggestions for what to order when eating out.

Chapter 6 encourages you to enjoy more home-cooked meals and gives you a collection of dozens of recovery recipes for everything from salad dressings and beverages to seafood and one-pot meals. Then chapter 7 offers an additional way to mend your health, with nutritional supplements.

There's lots to find out about food and recovery in the coming chapters, and good meals and good health ahead.

2 ALCOHOL AND AILMENTS

Why You Need to Eat Nutritious Foods

IF YOU NEED REASONS for eating nutritious foods, consider this: your body is probably crying out for them to repair the damage caused by alcohol. This chapter tells you about the many ways abusing alcohol can undermine health. Reading this plain-speaking information may make you feel uncomfortable if you've been downplaying to yourself the ill effects of your drinking or been ignoring health problems that alcohol may be exacerbating. But please keep reading: use this chapter to your advantage, as a reality check that can steer you in the right direction toward the foods you need to eat—foods that not only taste good but that will *help your body heal*.

Here, you'll probably come across some ailments that you already know you have, as well as perhaps other problems that deserve investigating with your doctor. Such health issues, if not addressed, can continue to undermine your well-being and vitality even as you maintain abstinence. But the good news is that the days and years ahead can be better than you may have imagined, in terms of your health, simply by your making the decision to improve your diet. Eating nourishing foods on a regular basis can reverse much of the harm that has been done and will have you feeling better surprisingly quickly.

So, how much damage can alcohol do? It is well known that alcoholism can lead to cirrhosis of the liver and that, for some people who continue to drink too much, cirrhosis can progress to liver failure and be fatal. But alcohol not only damages directly; it can also disrupt natural body processes significantly enough to increase the risk of a wide range of degenerative diseases. In fact, abusing alcohol can harm virtually every system, including cardiovascular, skeletal, and nervous systems. Of course, not everyone who has abused alcohol has a problem with all of these, but the functioning of at least one or another system in the body has likely been weakened to some degree.

The Not-Me Syndrome

In general, people who abuse alcohol know, at least somewhere deep down, that their drinking behavior is risky, but many think that for them drinking is risk free because the level of their drinking is "normal." They cling to the comforting stereotype of the sloshed drunk swinging from a lamppost and discount their own drinking behavior and the effect it may be having on their health if they do not fit that extreme stereotype.

In actuality, the amount of alcohol the body can safely handle is quite small. The federal Dietary Guidelines for Americans recommends up to one drink per day for women and up to two drinks per day for men (see page 28 for one reason why). These quantities are based on ethanol content, a standard drink providing a half ounce of ethanol per drink, the amount that an individual can typically metabolize in one hour. Consequently, one drink is equal to the following: a standard 12-ounce bottle of beer; one standard 1.5-ounce jigger of 80 proof distilled spirits, such as whiskey or rum; or a 5-ounce glass of wine, which is equal to a mere 10 tablespoons or a little more than $^1/_2$ cup.

Ailments at a Glance

If a whole chapter about the physical problems that can be caused by drinking too much is more than you can take right now, with the stress you may be under trying to maintain abstinence, just take a look at this list of ailments. It gives you a quick overview of the many health issues linked to alcoholism. If you want to get started on the Eating for Recovery program right away, jump ahead to chapter 3, which introduces the recovery foods.

Conditions that can result from alcohol abuse:

▶ Angina
▶ Brain degeneration
▶ Esophagitis, gastritis, ulcers
▶ Fatty liver and cirrhosis
▶ Decreased testosterone
▶ Greater susceptibility to infectious diseases, such as respiratory infections, pneumonia, and tuberculosis
▶ Heart disease
▶ Hypertension
▶ Hypoglycemia
▶ Increased risk of cancer of the upper digestive tract and liver
▶ Increased levels of triglycerides in the blood
▶ Muscle breakdown
▶ Nutrition-related problems, such as poor digestion and vitamin and mineral deficiencies
▶ Osteoporosis
▶ Pancreatitis
▶ Psoriasis
▶ Psychiatric disorders

Unfortunately, this isn't even the complete list. You're not alone if you were surprised by some of the items associated with alcoholism. Many people don't know that such disorders as thinning bones, lowered immunity, and even heart disease can be associated with drinking too much. Your body may well be in need of more help than you realize.

Alcohol's Path of Potential Destruction

How is it possible that alcohol can affect so many different areas of the body? Let's take a look at the route a drink takes as it enters the body and passes through the system.

Meet the Real Culprits

It's not the alcohol itself or, as chemists call it, *ethanol*, that does the damage, but acetaldehyde, a substance you may not even have heard of. This is the compound that results when the body metabolizes alcohol, a process that for the most part takes place in the liver. Acetaldehyde is highly toxic so the body quickly alters it, oxidizing it to become *acetate*. Normally, the acetate then breaks down into two harmless substances, carbon dioxide and water.

When intake of alcohol is low, the liver is able to handle the load of acetaldehyde produced so that it doesn't accumulate in the liver and blood and do harm. The process involves an enzyme, *alcohol dehydrogenase*, which the liver produces in sufficient quantity to handle a drink or two. But chronic consumption of high levels of alcohol is another matter, because an alternative means of metabolizing alcohol kicks in. This system is called the *microsomal ethanol-oxidizing system* (MEOS) and involves a more elaborate set of chemical reactions. The MEOS greatly enhances the conversion of alcohol to acetaldehyde. This chemistry also spews out *free radicals*, powerfully destructive atoms that react with anything they come in contact with, damaging cells and aging the body.

Acetaldehyde is also carcinogenic, interfering with the synthesis and repair of DNA, the part of the cell that directs reproduction. In addition, as the liver takes on the burden of detoxifying this compound, it is less able to shield the body from other carcinogens present in food and the environment.

First Stop: The Digestive Tract

It's estimated that one-third to one-half of individuals who abuse alcohol have gastrointestinal (GI) problems. Alcohol undermines the normal functioning of the digestive system in several ways:

▸ In the mouth, chronic alcohol abuse damages salivary glands and interferes with salivary secretion. It also increases the incidence of gum disease and tooth decay.

▸ Drinking too much can lead to inflammation of the esophagus, as well as acid reflux and heartburn. Damage to the lining of the esophagus also increases the risk of esophageal cancer.

▸ In the stomach, alcohol interferes with the secretion of gastric acid needed for the digestion of food. High doses of alcohol can injure the lining of the stomach, causing inflammation and possibly ulcers.

▸ In the intestines, alcohol disrupts normal muscle movement, shortening the time it takes for food to move through the intestinal track and pass from the body as waste. This can result in diarrhea, common for alcoholics.

▸ Both acute and chronic drinking can damage smooth muscle and the cells lining the intestine. This can limit the absorption of such nutrients as the B vitamins.

▸ Excessive drinking can cause an overgrowth of bacteria in the gut. In turn, this colonization may lead to malabsorption of food and nutrients and increased gut permeability. With this condition, also known as "leaky gut syndrome," large molecules of protein can enter the bloodstream and trigger an immune response, and toxins are now able to reach the liver and other organs where they can do damage.

▶ Alcohol interferes with the activity of such enzymes as lactase, which breaks down milk sugar, leading to an inability to digest dairy products.

▶ Alcohol can contribute to chronic inflammation of the pancreas, interfering with the absorption of fats and proteins. Although not part of the digestive system, the pancreas affects digestion because it produces enzymes that break down these components of food.

GI problems can occur even with a single dose of alcohol, but the good news is that the primary alcohol-related intestinal problems, diarrhea and malabsorption, can be eliminated by maintaining abstinence and returning to a normal diet.

Second Stop: The Liver

Once alcohol has passed through the digestive tract, it is rapidly transported to the liver, where blood vessels spread it throughout this organ as much as possible. Here, alcohol can potentially disrupt normal liver function. Although there is little risk with low intake, vulnerability rapidly increases as a person drinks more. All alcoholics display some signs of injury to the liver, and over 2 million Americans suffer from alcohol-related liver disease. Obesity—that is, being 30 percent above ideal body weight, which is increasingly common in today's society—is also an independent risk factor for alcoholic liver disease.

The demise of the liver happens in several fairly well defined stages:

Fatty liver. One of the primary tasks of the liver is to break down toxic compounds, such as alcohol. This process requires certain enzymes, substances that promote chemical reactions. Now, it happens that another important role of the liver is to metabolize fatty acids, a process that requires the same enzymes. When these enzymes are used up interacting with alcohol, and consequently fewer are available to break down the fatty acids, then fat deposits in liver tissue, hence fatty liver. This fat can also end up in the heart and arteries.

Alcoholic hepatitis. As fatty liver develops, the liver typically becomes inflamed and the result is alcoholic hepatitis. Symptoms are GI upset, loss of appetite, abdominal pain and tenderness, fever, jaundice, and mental confusion. Alcoholic hepatitis can be fatal if a person continues drinking but, if he or she abstains, the condition is often reversible. The hepatitis B and C viruses can also cause this condition. Consuming even small amounts of alcohol can be damaging to the liver for someone who is infected.

Cirrhosis of the liver. As hepatitis proceeds, the blood vessels in the liver become swollen and liver tissue becomes permanently damaged, with fibrous thickening of liver tissue, degeneration of cells, and severe scarring, a potentially fatal condition. Cirrhosis is not reversible but, with abstinence and adequate nourishment, chances of survival can increase and a person whose liver has begun this deterioration can restore a significant amount of liver function and health.

Frequently, patients with alcoholic liver disease have more than one of these conditions, such as fatty liver plus hepatitis, or hepatitis plus cirrhosis. In extreme cases, alcoholism can also lead to cancer of the liver and liver failure. Although the liver is an organ that can regenerate itself, severe liver damage is potentially fatal.

Fortunately, good nutrition can help repair liver damage. The recovery program presented in the following chapters is designed to do this. In addition, many of the special recovery foods recommended supply nutrients and other compounds that the liver needs to function normally. (See chapter 3, pages 52–58, for more about these.)

Third Stop: Almost Everywhere Else

The damage that alcohol can inflict on the body is not limited to the liver. Toxic compounds generated by the breakdown of alcohol also make their way to other areas in the system and cause trouble elsewhere. In addition, because the liver is an extraordinarily versatile organ and performs hundreds of different functions, when things go wrong with this organ, problems can show up in many other parts of the body.

The liver connection:

The cardiovascular system. The liver affects heart health by building and breaking down blood fats. It also makes the majority of cholesterol in the body and is the only organ able to remove cholesterol from the bloodstream. And because of its ability to assemble proteins, it produces clotting factors, which regulate the blood's ability to clot.

The immune system. The liver supports the immune system, producing antibodies that fight infection.

The skeletal system. Liver function impacts skeletal strength because vitamin D is metabolized in the liver and alcohol can disturb this process. Vitamin D is required for the absorption and transport of calcium and is involved in the modeling and remodeling of bone.

The pancreas. The liver assists the pancreas in steadying blood sugar levels by storing a form of sugar, glycogen, which it releases when needed to fuel muscle and other organs.

The digestive system. The liver supports digestive function by manufacturing bile, which is stored in the gallbladder and released into the small intestine, where it aids in the breakdown of fatty foods and promotes the absorption of fat-soluble vitamins. The liver also affects nutritional status by storing most of the iron in the body and keeping reserves of vitamin B_{12} and copper and 90 percent of the body's vitamin A.

The entire body. All areas of the body benefit from the liver's ability to filter more than one liter of blood every minute, removing toxins and microbes that might otherwise cause health problems.

The chemistry involved in liver function is indeed complex, and researchers are still exploring what's going on within the cells to learn more. What is quite clear is that many areas of the body may be adversely affected when the liver is damaged by alcohol. Making changes for the better in what you eat can help repair the liver and keep the damage from spreading.

Passing It Along

Fetal alcohol syndrome is one of the most well publicized and tragic consequences of drinking while pregnant. This results in infants with low birth weight, premature births, and physical and cognitive disabilities as well as behavioral problems later on. If you are pregnant or thinking about becoming a parent, it is literally vitally important to avoid alcohol. Your future child deserves to be healthy—and to be reared by a healthy parent, too.

Other Health Areas Affected by Alcohol

Excessive drinking can result in various chronic diseases, as well as less critical but still troublesome conditions such as an inability to handle stress and problems with sexual performance. The following gives you a list of health issues to watch out for.

Adrenal Burnout

With alcohol abuse, the adrenal glands produce less cortisol, a hormone that plays a key role in managing stress. Although abstaining from alcohol will help, a person who is abstinent may still have a lingering weakness in this area.

Sexual Function

While excessive intake of alcohol is likely to increase a person's interest in sex, it actually leads to sexual dysfunction. In men, alcohol abuse can cause a loss of sex drive, reduced fertility, and impotence. Levels of testosterone fall as estrogen increases. Drinking—in particular, binge drinking, which is commonly defined as, for women, four or more drinks on one occasion, and for men, five or more—suppresses the central nervous system, cutting off sensations. In women, alcohol lowers physiological arousal and raises estrogen levels. Women who abuse alcohol also are more prone to having menstrual problems, infertility, and an early menopause.

Heart Markers and What to Keep Checking

Homocysteine, an amino acid in the blood, is associated with an increased risk of heart attack, stroke, and peripheral artery disease. The liver plays a central role in the synthesis and metabolism of this compound. Chronic alcoholics, mainly those with liver damage, commonly have elevated levels of homocysteine. Elevated levels are found in people with fatty liver and cirrhosis. Even individuals only in the early stages of liver damage can have abnormally high levels.

Another marker for heart disease, *C-reactive protein* (CRP), also has a link to drinking. A 2007 study of college-age students conducted at the College of Saint Benedict in Saint Joseph, Minnesota, found that CRP levels rose sharply as drinking became heavier, evidence that excessive alcohol intake can set the stage for cardiovascular disease beginning even in these early years. See chapter 3, page 59, for information about CRP testing.

Heart Disease and Stroke

Light to moderate drinking has been getting a thumbs-up recently for its protective effect on heart health, although this remains a controversial subject. According to some research, light drinkers may have a healthier lifestyle and better eating habits than do heavier drinkers, accounting for their lower rates of heart disease. Then there's the question of who decides to drink. When a team of researchers at the University of Victoria in British Columbia and the University of California–San Francisco took a close look at fifty-four studies focusing on alcohol intake and health, they discovered that the great majority of these studies did not consider why abstainers chose not to drink in the first place. This opens the possibility that alcohol's apparent benefits are actually the result of comparing abstainers who had health problems and decided not to drink with drinkers who were already relatively fit.

What is certain is that heavy drinking is not good for the circulatory system. High intake raises blood pressure and increases the risk of arrhythmias, coronary heart disease, peripheral vascular disease, and stroke. According to the Institute of Alcohol Studies in England, if drinking does cut coronary heart disease risk, the amount needed for medicinal benefits isn't much. One drink every other day gives almost all the protection alcohol offers. More than two drinks a day increases your risk of heart disease, and the risk rises as intake increases.

Heavy drinking for at least ten years can cause a condition known as *alcoholic cardiomyopathy*: the heart becomes enlarged and the heart muscle can lose some of its ability to pump blood effectively. Women are especially susceptible to this condition, which often leads to heart failure.

Binge drinking comes with its own special risks: arrhythmias, an increased possibility of angina in those with heart disease, and increased risk of fatal heart attack. A study published in the *British Medical Journal* in 1997 concluded that binge drinkers were at a higher risk of heart attack and other major coronary events than were abstainers, even when overall volume of drinking was low.

Abusing alcohol, particularly binge drinking, which raises blood pressure, also increases the risk of stroke, the kind caused by a blood clot and, even more commonly, hemorrhagic stroke, caused by a burst vessel's bleeding into brain tissue. Even in young people, alcoholism is a risk factor for stroke. Besides abstinence, a heart-healthy diet can do much to prevent these conditions.

Glucose Intolerance and Diabetes

As many as 80 to 95 percent of alcoholics suffer from low blood glucose, or *hypoglycemia*. Hypoglycemia can occur after having a drink and can last as long as twelve hours. The symptoms of hypoglycemia are very similar to those of alcohol withdrawal—sweating, brain fog, blurred vision, confusion, headache, dizziness, hunger, anxiety, tremor, rapid heartbeat, and depression.

General glucose intolerance can persist for a period of time during abstinence until your body recovers, which unfortunately can put you at risk for relapse: low blood sugar creates a craving for anything that will rapidly raise the level of blood sugar, such as cookies, candy, a sugary cola—or an alcoholic drink. Many of the eating suggestions in the following chapters give you ways to make sure your blood sugar level remains under control.

Alcohol can also affect how the body handles sugar, by causing permanent damage to the pancreas, reducing its ability to secrete insulin, which results in type 1 diabetes. Frequent heavy drinking is also associated with type 2 diabetes, in which blood levels of both insulin and blood sugar are elevated. Alcohol coupled with already existing diabetes does extra harm, contributing to high blood pressure, elevated blood fats, and nerve damage.

Osteoporosis

Most research to date has focused primarily on heavy drinking in men, the results showing that most male alcoholics have some degree of osteoporosis. In the few studies that have taken a look at women's bone health as relating to alcohol, it appears that, at least in postmenopause, women have a lower risk than do men in the same age bracket. But in one large U.S. study, published in the *American Journal of Clinical Nutrition* in 1991, which involved over eighty thousand women between the ages of thirty-four and fifty-nine, those who took one to two drinks per day had a 133 percent increase in risk of hip fracture and a 38 percent increase for wrist fractures. In other research, part of the Framingham Study and published in the *American Journal of Epidemiology* in 1988, men who were heavy drinkers experienced almost ten times the number of hip fractures as did men who drank lightly. Of particular concern are adolescents who are heavy drinkers or who binge drink. Drinking during the years when peak bone mass normally forms can result in less initial bone mass and earlier onset of osteoporosis and related fractures.

How Alcohol Interferes with Bone Building

Current thinking is that alcohol has a direct effect on bone formation, reducing bone mass by interfering with the way bone remodels itself. Remodeling is a continuous process as mineral in bone is reabsorbed into the system while new mineral is deposited. With alcoholism, reabsorption proceeds while bone building slows. This can occur even when alcohol has caused no significant damage to the liver. The resulting loss of bone density happens gradually, closely tied to how long a person has been drinking and the quantity of alcohol consumed. Once you become abstinent, normal bone remodeling rapidly resumes in as little as two weeks, but how much bone mass was depleted while you were drinking remains a concern.

Building healthy bone requires a range of vitamins and minerals besides calcium. Many of the recommended foods in this book were chosen because they supply these nutrients. The recovery eating program is also protective because it minimizes such substances as refined sugars, white flour, and coffee. These foods acidify the system, triggering the body to buffer the acid with alkaline minerals, which are then drawn from the bones.

Degeneration of the Nervous System

Chronic drinking and, in particular, binge drinking, puts the brain at risk. Memory may be impaired and there may be problems with cognitive function and even dementia in extreme cases. In addiction, according to research sponsored by the National Institute on Alcohol Abuse and Alcoholism and published in *Alcohol Research and Health* in 2003, about half of the nearly 20 million alcoholics in the United States are thought to have some form of psychological problems ranging from mild to severe.

The Liver's Link to the Brain

When a person drinks more alcohol than the liver can readily detoxify, dangerous by-products of alcohol metabolism can pass through the nor-

---

The Alcoholic Brain Drain

Problems with thinking and mood associated with drinking appear in a predictable sequence, because alcohol first damages the outer areas of the brain before proceeding to the interior, and each section of the brain has specific functions.

▸ Damage to the outer brain causes inhibitions to drop. Euphoria sets in and judgment is distorted.
▸ When alcohol arrives at the cerebellum, coordination and perception decline and there's a risk of memory blackouts.
▸ Reaching the middle of the brain, alcohol impairs reflexes, and a person may experience confusion and/or stupor and even lapse into a coma.
▸ The final and fatal stage is when alcohol reaches the brain's inner core, the medulla. The heart stops and breathing ceases.

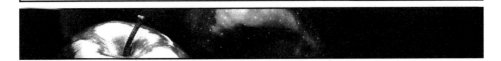

mally protective blood-brain barrier. In the brain, alcohol triggers inflammation and fluid retention and increases free radicals in brain tissue. Fewer healthy new nerve cells are formed to replace damaged ones. Consequently, brain activity slows, causing disruptions in normal thinking processes and changes in behavior and motor function.

When the liver is sluggish, its detoxification processes slow down and toxins accumulate. The toxin buildup can result in a person's having difficulty thinking clearly and waking up in the morning with "brain fog."

Prolonged liver dysfunction associated with fibrosis and cirrhosis can lead to hepatic encephalopathy, a condition that can result in cognitive, motor, and psychiatric problems. This condition can be fatal but may be reversible with adequate nutrition and hydration.

The brain requires thiamine, vitamin B_1, for normal functioning. Alcohol interferes with the body's absorption, storage, and use of this vital nutrient. A lack of thiamine can contribute to damage deep within the brain, leading to severe problems with cognition. Alcohol abuse, in extreme instances, can result in the condition known as Wernicke-Korsakoff syndrome. Malnourished alcoholics may develop this syndrome as poor eating habits increase the risk.

Alcohol as a Depressant

Alcohol also depletes hormones the brain produces that regulate mood. Specifically, alcohol lowers serotonin, known as the "feel-good" hormone. Although low doses of alcohol act as a stimulant, in fact, it is classified as a depressant. Drinking too much can bring on feelings of depression as well as anxiety and aggression. For individuals with mood and anxiety disorder, symptoms are likely to worsen even with moderate alcohol intake.

Immunity

One of the most overlooked medical complications of alcohol abuse is its effect on immunity. Abusing alcohol can affect the regulation of the immune system and disrupt its normal functioning, increasing susceptibility to such diseases as pneumonia and tuberculosis as well as less serious ailments, such as urinary tract infections.

The immune system fights infection with many different types of "warrior" cells, some of which the liver produces. Both chronic and binge drinking can reduce the effectiveness of these cells. A healthy diet that supplies such nutrients as zinc and vitamins A and C can help support an immune system impaired by alcohol.

Your Body Is Trying to Tell You Something!

Drinking too much may have left you with a weakness in one body function or another. If you've been in a recovery program or are working with a doctor to reestablish your health, you may already have been told where you need to put special focus. But if you haven't had the benefit of such advice, you can still have a good idea of what's gone wrong just by paying attention to what your body is saying. Typical health problems that crop up with alcoholism have the following common symptoms:

▸ *Low blood sugar:* sweating, anxiety, shakiness, racing heart, hunger pangs soon after eating something sugary, headache, brain fog, blurred vision, and/or depression
▸ *Impaired digestion:* gastritis, heartburn, and/or gum disease
▸ *Impaired liver function:* fatigue, brain fog, headaches, acne, psoriasis, and/or autoimmune and inflammatory disease

Whatever the particular ailment these symptoms may indicate, even in nondrinkers, these are signs that it's time to make sure you see a physician and have appropriate exams and lab tests—and that you're eating right. Fortunately, diet can play a powerful role in reversing these conditions.

Cancer

Alcoholism is a major risk factor for various cancers. The strongest link between alcohol and cancer is cancer of the upper digestive tract, including the esophagus, mouth, and throat. There's also a greater risk of stomach cancer, particularly in the upper portion of the stomach. While alcohol poses a lower risk of colon and rectal cancer, one study conducted at Northwestern University and published in the *Archives of Internal Medicine* in 2006 found that colon cancer patients with a history of both smoking and drinking contracted the disease eight years earlier than did patients who did not both smoke and drink.

Poor eating habits that result in nutrient deficiencies are another factor contributing to cancer risk. Research suggests that heavy drinkers are probably deficient in folic acid, iron, riboflavin, selenium, vitamin E, and zinc; these deficiencies may contribute to cancer development. They may also be lacking in beta-carotene, vitamin C, and the phytonutrients lutein and zeaxanthin, nutrients thought to help prevent cancer. Eating an abundance of fruits, vegetables, and other plant foods can replenish these and supply additional cancer-protective compounds as well.

Getting Short-Changed on Calories

Alcohol has 7 calories per gram, a sizable amount, less than a gram of fat but more than a gram of carbs. Calories are normally a source of energy for the body, but this may not be the case for someone abusing alcohol. Heavy drinking can shift the normal metabolism of alcohol to an alternative process that burns more of the calories that alcohol supplies. Combine this with scant food intake, and an alcoholic can end up low on fuel and even underweight (this is certainly *not* a recommended means of weight loss!).

Alcohol and Breast Cancer

Studies show a link between alcohol consumption and a modest increase in the risk of breast cancer, with a greater impact when intake is high. In research that combined results from six different studies, published in the *International Journal of Cancer* in 1991, women who consumed three or more drinks a day had a 69 percent higher rate of breast cancer than did nondrinkers. There's even evidence that having as few as one to two drinks a day can result in some increase in risk. However, not all studies show this close association, and more research is needed to give women guidance. What does seem to be fairly clear is that the risk of breast cancer rises as

---

Alcohol's Gender Bias

Alcohol is tougher on women than it is on men. Women feel more of an immediate effect than men do after drinking the same amount of alcohol. One reason for this is that a woman's body contains less water than does a man's. Alcohol is water soluble. A female drinker ends up with a higher concentration of alcohol in her system than does a man drinking the same amount, because her body is less able to dilute it. In addition, women produce less of the enzyme that breaks down alcohol into harmless substances.

Women also suffer a heavier physical toll from chronic alcohol abuse than men do: Women tend to become addicted faster and are more vulnerable to alcohol's ill effects on health. They are also likely to experience a quicker onset of alcohol-related health issues, such as cirrhosis of the liver, heart disease, and reproductive problems, as well as a decline in such mental functions as visual memory, spatial planning, and problem-solving. And, according to the Centers for Disease Control, in the "late stages" of alcoholism, women more quickly develop malnutrition.

greater amounts of alcohol are consumed, regardless of the source, whether wine, beer, or some form of distilled spirits.

How alcohol increases the risk of breast cancer may include such factors as:

▸ Drinking patterns

▸ Weight

▸ Use of supplemental hormones

▸ The health of a woman's immune system

▸ Family history of breast cancer

▸ Alcohol's effect on the chemistry within cells

Alcohol can raise estrogen levels, a risk factor for breast cancer, by increasing the conversion of precursor hormones to estrogen. Even as little as one drink a day can increase levels of this hormone, according to a study of postmenopausal women. An insufficient intake of fruits and vegetables, often a problem associated with drinking, can also be a factor. Research shows that women who eat the lowest quantities of these foods have a higher risk for breast cancer. Once again, here is evidence that eating wholesome foods is key to preventing disease.

Treating Ailments with Healing Recovery Foods

Using the recipes in this book, you can tailor your eating to particular conditions, as certain foods are especially beneficial for specific ailments. Take a look at the following chart. It matches recipes with health conditions, to help you get the most benefit from recovery eating. If you are already affected by or wish to prevent any of these ailments, help is on its way—in the form of delicious recovery foods!

HEALTH GOALS	HEALING DISHES
GOOD DIGESTION	MANGO LASSI *(page 286)*
	NEARLY INSTANT CURRIED "SQUASH" SOUP *(Menu 13, page 213)*
	KASHA WITH MUSHROOMS AND WALNUTS *(page 182)*
	YOGURT-BERRY SUNDAE *(Menu 11, page 167)*
	POACHED PEARS SCENTED WITH CARDAMOM *(Menu 19, page 276)*
NORMAL LIVER FUNCTION	SPINACH-EGG SCRAMBLE *(Menu 9, page 170)*
	GRILLED HALIBUT WITH TAPENADE *(Menu 18, page 237–238)*
	LENTILS WITH CARAMELIZED ONIONS *(page 190–191)*
	CARROTS WITH THEIR TOPS, MEDITERRANEAN-STYLE *(page 199)*
	SAUTÉED BRUSSELS SPROUTS *(page 203–204)*
BLOOD SUGAR CONTROL	HEALTHY BREAKFAST SHAKE *(Menu 7, page 124)*
	SPICED AND TOASTED NUTS *(page 266)*
	CREAMED HERRING ON WHOLE-GRAIN RYE BREAD *(Menu 8, page 128)*
	STEAK SALAD *(Menu 16, page 253)*
	FRUITY HERBAL TEAS *(page 285)*

HEALTH GOALS	HEALING DISHES
STEADY NERVES	COFFEE-SUBSTITUTE CAFE LATTE (*page 287*)
	TABBOULEH (*Menu 18, page 176*)
	WINTER SQUASH IN COCONUT MILK (*page 205*)
	TUNA FISH CAKES WITH SPICY MUSTARD MAYONNAISE (*page 230*)
	ORANGE AND WALNUT SALAD (*Menu 1, page 220*)
HEALTHY HEART	ROLLED OATS (*Menu 1, page 109*)
	BLACK BEAN PÂTÉ (*page 196–197*)
	SCALLOP SEVICHE WITH AVOCADO (*page 238*)
	TURKEY CHILI (*Menu 2, page 114*)
	WALNUT OIL DRESSING (*page 272*)
STRONG BONES	YOGURT CHEESE (*Menu 21, page 265–266*)
	COLD CEREAL AND FRUIT (*Menu 6, page 122*)
	PINTO BEANS WITH A MEXICAN ACCENT (*page 189*)
	GREEN BELL PEPPERS STUFFED WITH BROWN RICE AND SPICES (*page 177*)
	SALAD BAR MINESTRONE SOUP (*Menu 15, page 215*)

HEALTH GOALS	HEALING DISHES
HEALTHY BRAIN	SAVORY SALMON SANDWICH *(Menu 5, page 259)* WITH ASPARAGUS SOUP *(Menu 5, page 214)*
	TILAPIA TACO *(page 232)*
	MEXICAN GAZPACHO SOUP *(Menu 11, page 214–215)*
	BRAISED LEEKS *(page 201–202)*
	HOMEMADE BLUEBERRY SYRUP *(Menu 12, page 172–173)*
PREVENT CANCER	ARUGULA SALAD WITH CHICKPEAS, ARTICHOKES, AND ROASTED SWEET RED PEPPERS *(page 195–196)*
	GARLIC SHRIMP *(Menu 9, page 231)*
	STIR-FRIED BROCCOLI AND SHIITAKE MUSHROOMS *(page 206)*
	PASTA PRIMAVERA WITH PESTO *(Menu 6, page 183)*
	SALAD BAR STIR-FRY *(Menu 4, page 240–241)*

3 FOODS THAT HELP YOU REPAIR, RENEW, AND RECOVER

ACH PAGE IN THIS chapter is filled with offerings of great-tasting foods that can help repair the damage that alcohol can inflict on your body. You'll find various lists of these foods, arranged according to the benefits they offer. These ingredients, easy to incorporate into everyday meals, can help you make up for any vitamins and minerals missing in your diet or that have been mishandled by your body because of heavy drinking. These foods can help slow down and reverse the progression of such alcohol-related ailments as poor digestion, difficulty managing blood sugar, liver problems, osteoporosis, and cancer. This is medicine that works and is a pleasure to take.

A Quick Look at Eating for Recovery

There's an easy way to remember what kinds of foods can help you restore your health. They are the foods your grandmother would have recognized as being edible: fruits, vegetables, a chicken. Not some oversweetened, fake-flavored, foodlike substance in a box. Here are the chief characteristics of foods that need to be the mainstay of your meals.

Fresh. Fresh produce retains more of its original nutrients than does produce that has been frozen or canned before reaching your kitchen. Fresh fruits and vegetables deliver fiber as well as vitamins and minerals that can help you in the recovery process.

Unprocessed and unrefined. Unprocessed and unrefined foods are the mainstay of the recovery diet. They supply many vitamins and minerals that may become deficient with alcohol abuse. They also are likely to be free of the many chemical additives found in processed food products, which can burden the liver as it works to detoxify these substances.

Colorful. Many nutrients in food are actually pigments, the reason that tomatoes are red and blueberries are blue. Eating a range of colors, from red, orange, and yellow foods to those that are green or blue-purple, gives you a good mix of these phytonutrients (literally, "plant nutrients"), chemical compounds plants make that give them color, fragrance, and taste. Phytonutrients have many health benefits, including the ability to fight cancer. They are needed for recovery because, in our body, they function as antioxidants (which destroy dangerous free radicals), dampen inflammation (a topic covered later in this chapter), and otherwise strengthen the body's ability to detoxify harmful substances. Generally speaking, the brighter or deeper the color, the more nutritious the food: dark romaine lettuce packs in more nutrients than does the pale iceberg kind, for example.

Varied. When you eat an assortment of ingredients, you are more likely to benefit from a variety of nutrients. Don't have the same foods every day—become more adventurous. Have some oysters rather than tuna, and you'll be giving yourself a big dose of copper. Munch on a few Brazil nuts rather than peanuts, and you'll get your daily quota of selenium.

Organic. Give your liver a break and go organic. After all, this busy organ has already struggled enough, detoxifying all the alcohol that has come its way over the years. Lighten the load of pesticides that it also must break down, by starting to shop for organic ingredients. (If you don't like vegetables, discovering how good they taste without chemical sprays and preservatives might change your mind!) You can learn more about organic foods in chapter 4.

Variety in Name Only

The foods in the standard American diet, although they may sound varied enough, can be quite repetitive. Have a coffee shop breakfast of bacon and eggs, hash browns, and toast, along with some tomato ketchup, and then for lunch fix yourself a ham sandwich made with more bread and a piece of lettuce. Go to a restaurant for dinner and order steak and potatoes; while you're waiting for this to arrive, munch on the dinner roll and the lettuce and tomato salad. A day of eating like this gives you repeats of potatoes, pork, and the same few vegetables, plus wheat at all three meals.

To break the monotony, when you next go shopping, why not pick up berries and yogurt for breakfast, a can of salmon rather than canned tuna to make a sandwich for lunch, and a turkey breast and sweet potatoes to roast for dinner? Or, why not be even more adventurous and bake your own breakfast muffins, spark up your chicken salad with papaya and avocado, and then whip up a Turkish-style dinner of minted meatballs and flavorful rice pilaf plus ready-made exotic dips? Each time you enter a market, make a point of bringing home at least one healthy food or ingredient you have never tried before; for example, bring home some persimmons, Seckel pears in season, orange winter squash, broccoli rabe, fresh clams, buffalo meat, and mesquite-scented honey. Have some fun with all the fascinating foods out there and do some culinary exploring.

The Right Mix of Proteins, Fats, and Carbs

Eating for recovery features a moderate amount of each of the three major food components: proteins, fats, and carbohydrates. You won't be asked to go super high or low on any of these. Here's the general formula:

▶ 20 percent calories from protein

▶ 30 percent calories from fat

▶ 50 percent calories from carbohydrates

Protein—An Essential Component of Your *Body*

Alcohol interferes with the breakdown of food protein into amino acids, as well as with how the small intestine and liver process these amino acids. Alcohol also causes problems with the synthesis of amino acids back into those proteins your body is actually made of. In addition, both chronic and acute drinking increase the excretion of nitrogen, essential for building protein, resulting in a loss of lean tissue mass and skeletal muscle protein. Including sufficient protein in your diet can reverse the effects of liver disease. However, that doesn't mean a high-protein diet, like those prescribed for weight loss, is right for recovery, either. Keep serving sizes of meat and poultry to about 4 ounces. However, in case of cirrhosis of the liver, protein tolerance can vary considerably and has a small margin of safety, requiring close monitoring by a physician.

Fats—Quality, Not Just Quantity

For general health, keeping fat intake moderate is called for; this is particularly important when there is fatty infiltration of the liver, a condition seen in all active alcoholics and even in some nonalcoholics who drink moderately. A diet high in fat promotes fatty liver. What does a diet high in fat look like? It's a day's worth of eating that starts with bacon for break-fast and cream in your coffee, a wedge of pizza and an oily salad for lunch, and, at dinner, spare ribs followed by a scoop of ice cream for dessert. You might get away with having a reasonable portion of some of these foods at one meal, if you balance them with lean foods at the other two, but regu-larly eating this way loads you up with fat.

The other issue is what kind of fat you're selecting. To support the re-covery process, it's important to limit saturated fat, the kind found in red meat and butter. High intake of saturated fat also increases the risk of de-veloping fatty liver and blocks the flow of bile and toxins from the liver. Dip your bread into extra-virgin olive oil rather than spreading it with but-ter. Choose turkey over beef when ordering from a restaurant menu.

Are you surprised that so much fat is recommended in a healthy diet? The key is which kind: you do need to keep a good level of HDL ("good") cholesterol in your system, while lowering the LDL ("bad") kind. How can you do this? Replace some of the saturated fat in your diet with the mo-nounsaturated fats, the staple of the famous Mediterranean diet proven to be heart healthy. Food sources include olives, avocados, and almonds, as well as the cooking oils made from these. Such oils retain some of the fat-soluble vitamins, such as vitamin E, and minerals that were present in the original seed, fruit, or nut from which they were extracted, yet they don't contain residues of chemicals usually used in processing. Unrefined oils

Further Limiting Fat Intake

Depending upon the degree of injury your liver has suffered due to alco-hol, you should check with your physician about any further restriction of fats you may require at this particular time in your recovery process.

also contain fewer free radicals. In the refining process, oils may reach temperatures as high as 500°F, which generates the formation of these. Stock up on extra-virgin olive oil, an unrefined oil that is minimally processed; you can even cook and sauté with it as long as the temperature stays within a moderate range and is heated for only a brief period. Another unrefined oil that is widely sold in markets is unrefined safflower oil. Most of the recipes in this book call for either one of these two oils, staples of the recovery kitchen.

Polyunsaturated fats, those in vegetable cooking oils and fish, also have a place in recovery eating. You can read about these in chapter 4.

Carbs—Aim for Nourishing and Natural

The carbohydrates story is simple. Although carbs have been given a bad rap recently, this remaining 50 percent of calories, made up of starches and sugars, are also your allies in recovery—*if* you eat them in their whole, natural, unrefined, and unprocessed form. The primary foods that supply these are fruits and vegetables and whole grains, full of the many vitamins and minerals that are essential to replace after alcohol abuse. These healthy ingredients give you fiber as well.

Having sufficient carbohydrates in your diet may also help with abstinence. Carbs produce a feel-good fix because eating them increases the production of serotonin, a brain chemical that gives a person a feeling of well-being. When people in recovery don't have enough carbohydrates in their diet, they may turn to that other source of carbs—an alcoholic drink. During recovery, a need for carbs can also show up as a craving for sweets. Many people in recovery, as they first become abstinent, develop a sweet tooth, even though they probably didn't need sweets as much in their drinking days. While having a dessert is far preferable to having a drink, this isn't a license to binge on sugar whenever you wish. You may have a day when you can't stop yourself from indulging in starchy comfort foods or sweets, but the goal is to substitute whole-foods carbs—whole grains, vegetables, and fruits—rather than consuming their overly processed cousins. You'll find out more about the best kinds of carbs to eat on pages 44–46, where you'll learn about the methods of measuring the effect carbs have on blood sugar—the glycemic index and glycemic load.

Deciding Which Foods to Eat

If you've basically been relying on fast foods for most of your meals, or perhaps eating one decent meal a day but skipping the other two, just eating three meals a day and adding some fruits and vegetables and whole grains to your diet would already be a huge step to feeling better and a reason for congratulations. But don't stop there! The foods on the recovery menu are more fine tuned than that. They're nutrient-packed, life supporting, and targeted to help the body heal from the effects of alcohol. We're talking premium-grade eats. Why waste your time, money, and calories on anything else?

Replenishing Vitamins and Minerals

Some foods on the recovery menu have earned their place because they are especially good sources of certain vitamins and minerals that may be deficient as a result of alcohol abuse. Erratic eating habits, changes in appetite, and a tendency to use alcohol as a replacement for food can leave a person low in various nutrients.

Deficiencies also arise because of how alcohol affects the way a person's body handles foods and specific nutrients. As you learned in chapter 2, a damaged pancreas is less able to produce digestive enzymes, preventing food from being broken down and nutrients absorbed. A malfunctioning GI tract also impairs absorption of nutrients; and when the kidneys are affected by alcohol, the amount of nutrients excreted in the urine increases. As for specific nutrients, alcohol also inhibits the conversion of vitamin B_2, riboflavin, to its active form, and the process of detoxifying alcohol uses up zinc.

Researchers have identified many possible mineral and vitamin deficiencies in those who drink. Minerals that can become depleted include calcium, iron, magnesium, selenium, and zinc. Possible vitamin deficiencies are the fat-soluble vitamins—vitamins A, D, E, and K; the water-soluble B vitamins, including vitamins B_1 (thiamine), B_2 (riboflavin), B_6, B_{12}, folic acid, and niacin; and vitamin C.

Of course, it won't do any harm if you simply eat all the foods that supply these vitamins and minerals, even if you don't know precisely which ones you most need. In wholesome natural foods, nutrients come ready-mixed in the right combinations and proportions and you get all those that have been identified, plus those still waiting to be discovered. Nutritional supplements can only give you so much support; they can never fully make up for nutrient-poor ingredients and haphazard eating. These key foods are also the basis of a generally healthy diet. To help you get started eating these foods at your very next meal, here is a handy list of each mineral and vitamin, along with the foods that provide them. The focus is on common ingredients to make it easy for you to shop and to begin including these nutrients in your meals. In general,

---

Getting a Vitamin and Mineral Checkup

Knowing if you have particular vitamin and mineral deficiencies can guide you to the foods you especially need to eat for recovery. But this takes more than guesswork. It's worth the time and effort to have your nutrient status assessed by a knowledgeable health professional. You can ask your doctor to order lab tests that measure nutrient levels and you might also want to consult with a nutritionist who can use a computer program to assess what you've been eating, to identify nutrients missing in your meals.

the items on the lists start with the most abundant sources of each vitamin or mineral.

MINERALS

Magnesium: nuts and seeds (such as cashews, almonds, and sesame seeds); green vegetables (such as spinach); whole grains (such as brown rice); seafood (such as shrimp and tuna); legumes (such as peanuts, navy beans, black-eyed peas, and lentils); bananas; dates

Zinc: seafood (such as oysters, sardines, and crab); meat (such as beef, dark-meat chicken, turkey, lamb, and pork); nuts (such as cashews); eggs; legumes (such as peanuts, green peas, and lima beans); turnips; parsley; grapes; garlic; fresh ginger; whole grains (such as rye and oats)

Selenium: Brazil nuts; seafood (such as oysters, salmon, and herring); meat (such as beef, pork, and chicken breast); whole grains (such as whole wheat and barley); eggs

Calcium: dairy foods (such as milk and yogurt); seafood (such as canned sardines and salmon with bones); dark leafy greens (such as collard greens and kale); legumes (such as great northern, kidney, and pinto beans); sweet potatoes; okra; acorn squash; oranges

Iron: clams; beef; legumes (such as lentils and kidney beans); raisins; nuts and seeds (such as almonds, cashews, and pumpkin and squash seeds); lettuce; parsley; beet greens; broccoli; strawberries; eggs

THE B VITAMINS

Thiamine: pork; tuna; nuts and seeds (such as sunflower and sesame seeds, pistachio nuts, and Brazil nuts); watermelon; whole grains (such as oatmeal, whole-grain rye, and brown rice); legumes (such as lentils and pinto and black beans)

Riboflavin: dairy products (such as yogurt and milk); beef; oysters; nuts (such as almonds and hazelnuts); whole grains (such as whole wheat, bulgur, and wild rice); mushrooms; asparagus; dark greens (such as beet greens and spinach)

Vitamin B$_6$: seafood (such as tuna, bluefish, orange roughy, and bass); watermelon; bananas; potatoes and sweet potatoes; meat (such as light meat chicken, beef, and pork); flaxseeds

Vitamin B$_{12}$: seafood (such as clams, oysters, sardines, bluefish, salmon, flounder, and tuna); beef; lamb; dairy products (such as Swiss cheese, yogurt, milk, cottage cheese, and blue cheese); eggs

Folate (folic acid): whole grains (such as barley and brown rice); legumes (such as peanuts, black-eyed peas, chickpeas, and lentils); papayas; oranges; asparagus; spinach; beets; avocados; walnuts

OTHER VITAMINS

Vitamin A and beta-carotene: red, orange, or yellow produce (such as sweet potatoes, carrots, butternut and Hubbard squash, red leaf lettuce, mangoes, cantaloupe, red bell pepper); kale; parsley; eggs; chicken; seafood (such as tuna, mackerel, and herring)

Vitamin C: papaya; citrus fruits (such as oranges and grapefruit); mangoes; cantaloupe; strawberries; parsley; bell peppers; broccoli; red cabbage; romaine lettuce

Vitamin D: seafood (such as salmon, sardines, catfish, mackerel, herring, tuna, shrimp, and flounder); chicken; mushrooms; sunflower seeds; eggs; fortified milk

Vitamin E: nuts and seeds (such as sunflower seeds and oil and almonds); peanuts; seafood (such as cod, shrimp, and herring); butternut squash; asparagus; whole grains (such as whole wheat and rye); mangoes; bananas; eggs; extra-virgin olive oil

Vitamin K: dark leafy greens (such as kale, turnip greens, and spinach); lettuce; Brussels sprouts; parsley; broccoli; avocados; pistachio nuts; oats; green tea

Foods That Target Specific Ailments

The natural, fresh foods recommended here can give you more get-up-and-go and keep you feeling better in general. But you can also choose

---

The Low-Down on Liver

Beef and calf's liver are extraordinarily rich sources of many of the nutrients that alcohol abuse can diminish, including folate, iron, riboflavin, selenium, vitamins A, B_6, B_{12}, D, and zinc. Chicken livers are also a good source of many of these nutrients. However, liver has its downside, since its function is comparable to the oil filter in a car, collecting all sorts of toxins and unwanted substances. When you have this meat for dinner, your own liver must deal with what has accumulated in the animal's liver, as well. Particularly in the early stages of recovery, when your liver is most likely in need of repair, avoid eating this organ meat and rely on the many other sources of these nutrients. Then, later on, if you do crave a savory piece of liver topped with perhaps some sautéed onions, be absolutely sure to eat only liver that is organic so you don't also end up with pesticides, antibiotics, and growth hormones on your dinner plate.

foods that target a particular body function that may need some repairing because of heavy drinking. As you read in chapter 2, excessive intake of alcohol over time can lead to problems of the digestive system, impaired liver function, difficulties managing blood sugar, and even changes in the way the brain performs. Of these conditions, a problem with blood sugar is perhaps the easiest to remedy with food and the treatment that produces the quickest results. Let's first take a look at foods that help with this ailment.

Foods That Keep Blood Sugar Levels Steady

Problems with blood sugar are common among former alcoholics. If you usually get a rush of energy and then a drop after eating something starchy or sugary, you probably need to pay attention to how your body handles sugar. Dips in blood sugar can increase the craving for alcohol. In a study published in the *Journal of the American Dietetic Association* in 1991, when hospitalized patients with alcoholism restricted their sugar intake, their cravings for alcohol declined and they had significantly fewer hypoglycemic symptoms. It may be that the low blood sugar triggers the stress response and the impulse to drink. Fortunately, blood sugar levels respond quickly to changes in food choices. It just takes knowing which foods have the greatest impact on blood glucose.

Glycemic Index and Glycemic Load

Researchers have tested hundreds of specific foods to assess their effect on blood sugar. The measures they use to rank foods are called the *glycemic index* and *glycemic load*. The glycemic index (GI) usually takes white bread as the standard and assigns it a GI value of 100; other foods rank higher or lower. The GI of a particular food depends upon the amount of carbohydrate it contains and how fast the body is able to digest and absorb it. Once you understand this, it's easy to figure out that a glass of orange juice, which is very sweet and quickly absorbed into the system, will have a higher glycemic index than a fibrous stalk of raw broccoli, which is not sweet and takes time to digest. But the GI of some foods isn't as easy to estimate. For instance, it may surprise you that the natural sugars in fruit have less of an effect on blood sugar than does white table sugar, and that the GI of bagels is sky high.

Being aware of the GI of certain foods can be very helpful in making food choices, but the index does have one drawback: it doesn't factor in serving size. So in 1997, researchers at Harvard University introduced a more useful guide, the glycemic load (GL), which does consider serving size. Carrots' GI rating of 68 is only applicable if you plan to eat seven carrots at one sitting—not likely. Based on a more normal portion of *one* carrot, this favorite root vegetable now earns a much more acceptable GL rating of 3.

A slice of white bread just over 1 ounce in weight has a GL of 10. Generally, foods with ratings under 10 per serving are fine to eat. They won't increase the risk of type 2 diabetes, a possible complication of alcoholism. But many starchy foods top the standard measure of 10 by a long shot. Take a look at this chart for a comparison of the glycemic load of common foods, based on typical serving-size quantities. Note that protein and fat contain little or no carbohydrate and have a GL of 0.

FOOD ITEM	GLYCEMIC LOAD
BAGEL, 3$\frac{1}{3}$ OUNCES	34
WHITE RICE, 1 CUP, 6$\frac{1}{2}$ OUNCES	28
WHITE BREAD, 2 SLICES OR 2$\frac{3}{4}$ OUNCES	26
BAKED POTATO, 1 MEDIUM-SIZE, 5 OUNCES	26
WHOLE WHEAT BREAD, 2 SLICES OR 2$\frac{3}{4}$ OUNCES	23
FRENCH FRIES, 5 OUNCES	22
SWEET POTATO, 1 MEDIUM, 5 OUNCES	17
SWEET CORN, 3 OUNCES	7
APPLE, 4 OUNCES	6
KIDNEY BEANS, 5 OUNCES	6
LENTILS, 5 OUNCES	5

FOOD ITEM	GLYCEMIC LOAD
WATERMELON, 4 OUNCES	4
GREEN PEAS, 3 OUNCES	3
TABLE SUGAR, 1 ROUNDED TEASPOON, 1/6 OUNCE	3
PEANUTS, 1 3/4 OUNCES	2
STRAWBERRIES, 4 OUNCES	1
CHICKEN, 3 OUNCES	0
SALMON, 3 OUNCES	0
BACON, 1/2 OUNCE	0

For information on where to find complete listings of common foods and their glycemic index and glycemic load figures, see Recommended Reading on page 308.

Foods That Help—and Harm—Digestion

As you read in the preceding chapter, alcohol can cause problems all along the digestive tract. Acid reflux, inflammation of the lining of the stomach

---

The Glycemic Link to the Liver

White flour as well as sugars, such as high-fructose corn syrup, which pervade the food supply and are present in a vast array of products from colas, soups, and crackers to "honey-baked" hams, can do their part in undermining recovery, according to a recent study conducted by Children's Hospital Boston. Consuming these foods can lead to fatty liver disease. The researchers also concluded that eating a low-glycemic diet, one with relatively less effect on blood sugar, can prevent fatty liver disease.

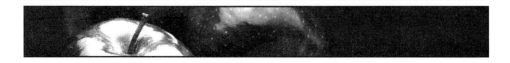

or gastritis, overgrowth of bacteria in the small intestine, and diarrhea are some of the ailments that can occur. Fortunately, abstinence resolves many of these problems and eating a selection of the right foods further promotes healing. Be careful though: while some foods can heal, others can aggravate problems.

Acid Reflux

Having a drink can trigger an episode of acid reflux, which happens when gastric juices move upward into the esophagus. What's happening is that the alcohol has relaxed the muscle between the stomach and esophagus that normally prevents such a backup. Changing your eating habits can help, with smaller meals recommended. A smaller meal causes less distention of the stomach, a trigger for acid reflux. Having an early dinner is also a good idea, so the stomach is likely to have already sent the meal in the right direction by bedtime. Lying down with a full stomach can bring on acid reflux.

A Chocolate Truffle for Dessert

On the glycemic load chart, did you happen to spot those high numbers for plain white rice, potatoes, and bagels? They earn such high rating because they are digested so quickly. But here's the good news: although a regular serving of such starchy foods will significantly add to your glycemic intake, a small amount of sugar will have a relatively lesser effect on your blood sugar. This means that you probably won't risk upsetting your blood sugar control very much by having a lovely mouthful of a sweet at the end of a meal. Chocolate truffles are a great choice because they're small and come with some fat to slow absorption. Or enjoy some of your favorite dessert. Just make sure to stop after a bite or two. Sharing the dessert with others can help your resolve!

Here is a list of foods and beverages that have been known to increase symptoms and so should be avoided:

▶ Fatty foods

▶ Chocolate

▶ Peppermint

▶ Acidic beverages, such as coffee, tea, and citrus juices

▶ Carbonated beverages

▶ Milk

▶ And of course, alcohol

Milk—A Mixed Blessing

Milk shows up on several of the food lists in this chapter, sometimes as a recommended food, other times with a warning. Indeed, milk has its virtues but it can also cause problems. It's an excellent source of calcium, as well as a source of vitamin D and B vitamins, and a handy source of protein. But it's one of the most common food allergens and can cause digestive stress in individuals who are lactose intolerant. Dairy products can also disrupt the bacterial flora in the gut. Some people "got milk," as the advertising slogan goes, but for others, milk's got them. If you find your body doesn't tolerate dairy foods, especially if your digestive tract needs repair because you have a history of drinking, milk is not for you. Soy or rice dairy substitutes that have been enriched with nutrients offer an alternative without the gastric distress.

Gastritis

Acute gastritis, causing abdominal pain, is associated with heavy drinking. Chronic gastritis in alcoholics is primarily due to infection with *Helicobacter pylori*, also the cause of ulcers. While this condition heals rapidly with abstinence, paying attention to what you're eating can also help.

Healing foods include those that supply antioxidants, such as beta-carotene, vitamin C, and zinc (see the list on pages 53–54). Ingredients that are anti-inflammatory can also be helpful (see page 58). There's also some evidence that chile peppers can protect against alcohol-induced gastritis. Their active ingredient, capsaicin, the pungent compound in cayenne, may help by increasing the flow of blood to the stomach.

In contrast, certain foods can irritate the stomach lining and should be avoided to prevent and treat this condition:

▸ Beverages containing caffeine, such as coffee, tea, and hot chocolate

▸ Decaffeinated coffee

▸ Acidic juices, such as pineapple and tomato juice

▸ Carbonated drinks

▸ Milk

▸ Salt

In addition, learning what could trigger any food sensitivities you may have and avoiding those foods may result in relief. See pages 88–89 for a list of symptoms of food sensitivity.

Overgrowth of Intestinal Flora

While the small intestine is normally relatively free of bacteria, changes in gut function due to alcohol can lead to an overgrowth of bacteria and thus, to a variety of digestive problems. As explained in chapter 2, these bacteria produce toxins that, once absorbed into the system, can make their way to the liver and cause damage to this organ already under attack from the alcohol itself. Drinking also makes it more likely that these toxins will be absorbed because ingesting alcohol increases the permeability of the intestinal wall.

Increase your intake of fiber. To restore healthy gut flora, eat more high-fiber foods. Fiber content is highest in whole grains, but moderate amounts of fiber are also found in fruit and vegetables, especially those eaten with their skin. Conversely, foods that promote overgrowth of gut flora are refined and low/lacking in fiber. These include refined sugars, such as white table sugar and high-fructose corn syrup, and white flour.

To add fiber to your diet, eat more of these foods:

▸ *Vegetables:* artichokes, avocados, broccoli, Brussels sprouts, cabbage, carrots and other root vegetables, cauliflower, corn, green beans, onions, potatoes with their skin, pumpkin, winter squash

▸ *Fruit:* apples, pears, peaches, and plums with their skins; bananas; blueberries and raspberries; oranges; dates

▸ *Legumes:* beans, lentils, peanuts, peas

▸ *Whole grains:* brown rice, bulgur, cracked wheat, oatmeal, whole wheat

▸ *Nuts:* almonds with their skins, walnuts

Say yes to yogurt. Being a fermented food, yogurt is a source of live, friendly bacteria that can reestablish normal flora in the gut. These microorganisms facilitate the digestion of fats and protein, the metabolism of hormones, including estrogens, and the production of vitamin K and certain B vitamins (folic acid, riboflavin, and vitamins B_5, B_6, and B_{12}), which can be deficient in people who drink too much. These bacteria also improve immune function.

When shopping for yogurt, be aware that all commercial brands of yogurt are not equal when it comes to bacterial content. First, make certain that the label states that the product contains "active cultures," or "live cultures"; and second, absolutely avoid "heat-treated" products, because bacteria cultures are destroyed during heat treatment. Also check which strains a given

The Option of Probiotic Supplements

If you know you have digestive problems, you may also want to take a probiotic supplement, since not all yogurt products deliver sufficient amounts of microorganisms and there's no way to tell how much you're getting. You can find out more about probiotics in chapter 7.

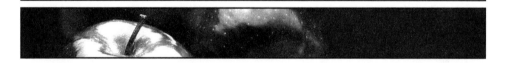

Friendly Carbs That Increase Friendly Bacteria

Fructo-oligosaccharides (FOSs) are carbohydrates, found in a range of foods, which encourage the growth of healthful bacteria (bifidobacteria and Lactobacillus acidophilus, the two strains also present in yogurt). Consuming FOSs can help reestablish a balance of flora in the intestines. FOS-containing foods include asparagus, bananas, barley, chicory, garlic, honey, onions, rye, and tomatoes.

product contains. You want the ingredient list to contain bifidobacteria and Lactobacillus acidophilus. (Another source of acidophilus is acidophilus milk, available in the dairy section of many markets.)

Diarrhea

An episode of acute diarrhea triggered by alcohol abuse calls for replacing liquids and calories and replenishing sodium and potassium. Have a glass of orange juice to give yourself a dose of potassium and make sure to salt your food for extra sodium. To treat acute diarrhea, you can also follow the BRAT diet. The letters stand for *b*ananas, *r*ice, *a*pples, and *t*oast—foods that are bland, easy to digest, and low in fiber. The restricted BRAT diet is for short-term use over a few days as recuperation begins.

Common foods can also cause diarrhea in people who are sensitive to them. Coffee is a frequent trigger. Fruit juice and the sugar substitute sorbitol can cause the intestines to hold water, leading to diarrhea. Also, if you are allergic to dairy foods or lactose intolerant, consuming dairy products may produce an upset stomach. See chapter 4 to find out more about food allergies and intolerances.

(If diarrhea continues for more than a few days, see a doctor, as this may indicate a more serious health condition.)

Impaired Liver Function

What you choose to eat can help the liver repair itself and restore normal function. The following foods should be restricted:

▸ *Saturated fats:* These should be limited, since this form of fat contributes to fatty infiltration of the liver.

▸ *Refined sugar:* A substance devoid of nutrients, this also should be cut to a minimum.

▸ *Beef or calf's liver:* These meats may come with an accumulation of toxic substances that will place extra stress on your liver (see page 43).

For optimal liver health, the focus should be on nutritional elements, such as antioxidants, fiber, and phytonutrients, which play a role in the way the liver detoxifies various substances, and on organic foods.

Detoxification. One of the primary functions of the liver is to break down and deactivate harmful substances and send them on their way out of the body. This process of detoxification happens with a one-two punch. In the first phase, harmful substances are converted to intermediary compounds. In the second phase, these compounds are then deactivated. But there's a potential problem. This chemistry needs to proceed on schedule because the intermediary compounds generated in phase one are often much more chemically active and therefore more toxic than the original substances. Efficient detoxification requires that you have enough of the right foods and nutrients to make sure that both phase one and phase two proceed on schedule.

Some of the foods that activate phase one detoxification are oranges, tangerines, and brassica-family vegetables: broccoli, Brussels sprouts, and cabbage. Phase two activators also include the brassica vegetables as well as caraway seeds and dill seeds, citrus peel, and fish oils. No, you don't have to eat all the rind on an orange, but you can add thin strips of lemon and orange zest to fruit compotes, salads, and pilafs for flavor and as a garnish.

Because this two-stage chemistry generates harmful free radicals, the detox process also increases your need for antioxidants, which can stop these free radicals from damaging tissues. Here's a list of some excellent food sources of antioxidants:

▸ *Beta-carotene:* butternut and Hubbard squash, cantaloupe, carrots, mangoes, parsley, red bell peppers, spinach, sweet potatoes

▸ *Vitamin C:* citrus, guava, papaya, sweet peppers

▸ *Vitamin E:* almonds, sunflower seeds, sweet potatoes, whole grains

▸ *Selenium:* Brazil nuts, brown rice, chicken, shrimp, whole wheat

▸ *Zinc:* cashews, duck, mushrooms, oysters

Special Nutrients in Plant Foods

Here's one more reason to eat more foods from the plant kingdom. Plant foods offer special phytonutrients that play key roles in detoxification processes. Researchers have identified many of these. Take a look at these powerful edible allies that can go to work for you!

Alpha-lipoic Acid

What it does. destroys harmful, free radical by-products of detoxification processes

Food sources. broccoli, Brussels sprouts, peas, potatoes, red meats, spinach, tomatoes

Glucosinolates, Such as Sulforaphane and Indoles

What they do. help the liver to detoxify chemicals, drugs, and pollutants

Food sources. cruciferous vegetables, such as broccoli, Brussels sprouts, cabbage, cauliflower, and especially broccoli sprouts (sprouted broccoli seeds)

Glutathione

What it does. facilitates the removal of fat-soluble toxins and acts as a powerful antioxidant—this is a vitally important compound.

Fighting Chronic Inflammation: Calling on the Culinary Fire Brigade

Another way alcohol undermines health is by promoting inflammation. In the process of metabolizing alcohol, liver cells produce small proteins, called *cytokines*, which rev up the immune system and trigger inflammation. The

---

Special Nutrients in Plant Foods *continued*

Food sources. asparagus, avocados, cantaloupe, cooked fish and meat, okra, oranges, peaches, potatoes boiled in their skins, raw spinach, strawberries, walnuts, watermelon

Inulin

What it does. lessens the detox burden on the liver by stimulating the kidneys and clearing out poisons produced by harmful bacteria in the gut

Food sources. artichokes, Jerusalem artichokes, raisins

Limonene

What it does. aids the liver in breaking up and transforming toxins for elimination

Food sources. lemon peel, mandarin orange peel, orange peel, and, to a lesser extent, the juice of these fruits

Sulfur Compounds

What they do. fuel certain detox processes that transform and thereby inactivate hormones, neurotransmitters, and drugs

Food sources. beans, broccoli, Brussels sprouts, egg yolks, garlic, onions, sweet red peppers

---

problem is that with habitual drinking, cytokine levels stay high and inflammation becomes chronic. This fire can spread beyond the liver, because when inflammatory immune cells are stirred up in one location, they can travel throughout the body. Such inflammation is now thought to be a factor in heart disease, obesity, cancer, and diabetes. It also plays a role in the development of conditions closely related to alcoholism, such as hepatitis and gastritis. (Any ailment that ends in "itis," such as arthritis and gingivitis, involves inflammation.)

Anti-inflammatory Foods

Fortunately, there are many tasty foods that can effectively turn down the heat. We're talking garlic and onions! Also, foods from both the land and the sea contain substances that reduce inflammation, counteracting inflammatory processes in a variety of ways. Some supply antioxidants that react

---

Getting in the Way of Detox

While many substances support the liver in cleansing the system, some trip up this organ's two-step detox process, inhibiting phase one chemistry. This is true of certain medications, such as antihistamines, benzodiazepines, and drugs that block stomach acid secretions (used to treat stomach ulcers). These drugs contain compounds that deactivate this first step. If you're taking medications, including over-the-counter preparations, ask your physician or pharmacist whether they contain such substances.

Grapefruit as well as its juice contain naringenin, a flavanone that causes this fruit to have the same effect—a reason to avoid grapefruit and its juice if you're in the first stages of withdrawal from alcohol and in the process of detoxifying. Grapefruit can also interfere with the effectiveness of some medications.

---

with free radicals, an inflammatory by-product of alcohol metabolism, and put these out of action. Fatty fish provide special oils that the body uses to build powerful anti-inflammatory compounds.

Additional Detox Support

Increasing Bile Flow

Any substance that promotes the flow of bile also supports detoxification. A nutrient or some other factor such as an amino acid that promotes this cleansing flow is described as *lipotropic*.

Lipotropic agents. Include some familiar vitamins such as vitamins B_6 and B_{12}, and folate, often deficient in alcoholics. (You'll find food sources of these on page 42.) Other lipotropic agents are the amino acid methionine, widely available in the diet, in protein foods that include cottage cheese, pork chops, and sea bass; choline, present in egg yolk and whole grains; and betaine, which is found in beets.

Such lipotropic foods also deliver an extra benefit, in that they promote the flow of fat to and from the liver. For this reason they are also useful in the treatment of fatty liver disease, hepatitis, and cirrhosis.

Soluble fiber. Also promotes increased bile secretion. Here are some high-soluble-fiber foods:

▶ *Fruit:* apples, apricots, bananas, oranges, peaches, pears, plums, prunes, strawberries
▶ *Legumes:* beans, lentils, peas
▶ *Nuts and seeds:* Brazil nuts, sesame seeds
▶ *Vegetables:* beets, broccoli, Brussels sprouts, cabbage, carrots, chicory (salad greens), green beans, okra, potatoes, spinach, sweet potatoes, tomatoes
▶ *Whole grains:* barley, brown rice, oats

Make a habit of including these anti-inflammatory ingredients in your meals, and you'll be taking an important step in preventing disease:

▸ Fruits and vegetables that are colorful, a sign they contain antioxidants: blackberries, blueberries, bell peppers (red, orange, yellow, or green), carrots, cranberries, raspberries, strawberries, and winter squash, to name a few

▸ Citrus fruits, such as oranges and lemons, which are an excellent source of the antioxidant vitamin C

▸ Whole grains and nuts that deliver the antioxidant vitamin E

▸ Sources of quercetin, an anti-inflammatory phytonutrient: broccoli, garlic, onions, and russet potatoes

▸ Herbs and spices such as chamomile, ginger, and rosemary

▸ Foods that contain anti-inflammatory fats: flaxseeds, free-range meats and poultry, seafood (such as salmon, mackerel, sardines, and tuna), walnuts, and wild game. (Chapter 4 tells you more about these fats on pages 78–81.)

Foods That Trigger Inflammation

Many of the foods that make up the standard American diet are pro-inflammatory, either because they contain substances that promote inflammation or because the person eating a particular food has an allergic reaction or doesn't tolerate that food, which in turn triggers the inflammatory reaction. The list of these foods includes the usual suspects:

▸ Refined white flour

▸ Sugar

▸ Red meat

▶ Dairy products

▶ Highly processed foods

▶ Food additives

▶ Foods that may trigger an allergic reaction or be difficult to tolerate: peanuts, eggs, milk, wheat, yeast, corn, soy, onions, citrus, berries, melon, chocolate, beef, pork, fish, and shellfish

---

Testing for Inflammation

If you are wondering whether your body is dealing with chronic inflammation, you can ask your doctor to give you a C-Reactive Protein (CRP) lab test. Be sure to request the "high-sensitivity" C-Reactive Protein test, new and inexpensive but not currently part of routine lab work. The more common CRP test that measures only sedimentation rate of red blood cells won't give you the information you need.

The Heat in Meat

Red meat contains arachidonic acid, which promotes inflammation. Beef contains the most, with pork and lamb about half as much. As for chicken, it's comparable to pork and lamb. Other protein foods, eggs and dairy, also contain some arachidonic acid, but the amount is far lower than in red meat. Free-range meats and poultry are also less inflammatory. Animals are fed on natural vegetation, which contains anti-inflammatory fats, and these end up on your plate.

In addition, any foods that cause a rapid rise in blood sugar can promote inflammation in individuals who are especially sensitive to this, such as those with type 2 diabetes.

This is not to say that none of the ingredients so typical of the modern diet should ever reach your lips. It's just a question of balancing anti-inflammatory foods with those that are pro-inflammatory. For instance, cooking oils, such as sunflower oil, corn oil, and soybean oil, can do their share in triggering inflammation when not balanced with complementary oils, such as fish oils, that dampen inflammation. Making sure to have a healthy balance of these in the diet is one of the goals of this nutrition program. You can read more about this in chapter 4, on pages 78–81.

Putting All This Good Eating Advice into Action

The foods featured in this chapter are powerful allies for your recovery. When deciding what to eat, remember to include these in your meals. Also consider any special needs you have, such as balancing your blood sugar, improving your digestion, reducing inflammation, detoxifying, avoiding foods to which you are allergic or intolerant, or perhaps just making up for deficient nutrients. Refer to the sections on special ailments and start having more of the targeted foods that remedy these conditions.

You may not be eating these recommended foods often, or at all. If you're not accustomed to eating fruits and veggies regularly, carry an apple with you to work or some cut up carrot sticks and sweet peppers as a snack. And when you go out and about, bring along a bag of almonds, walnuts, or sunflower seeds, or a mix of all three, for a quick anti-inflammatory fat/protein/nutrient hit.

To jump-start your recovery eating, you can also simply refer to the core list of recovery foods, which you'll find at the end of chapter 4 (on page 98). It's a collection of the foods that, in general, can do the most good for your health—star ingredients that deserve to be eaten regularly. They are featured in the recovery nutrition program that you'll read about next.

4 THE GOALS OF RECOVERY EATING

However you've been eating until now, you can always choose to eat a little better and the nutritional program for recovery gives you an easy way to start. This chapter presents the goals of the program, which are designed to help you transition gradually into consuming healthier foods. Improved nutrition happens one decision at a time. You reach for this, you don't reach for that; you replace a food that is highly refined and processed with one that is more natural; you switch from an item devoid of nutrients to another loaded with vitamins and minerals. You can start making such changes with your very next meal.

Plan a trip to the supermarket and bring some recovery ingredients home. Having the right ingredients on hand makes it more likely you'll put together recovery meals. And don't worry, recovery eating doesn't necessarily mean that you'll need to do lots of fussing in the kitchen. In the next chapter, you'll find many suggestions for what I call "go-togethers," rather than recipes, as simple as cooking pasta and then topping the pasta with prepared spaghetti sauce. You can see signs of this quick-fix meal prep everywhere in markets these days. Ready-made, precooked, precut, sliced and diced ingredients and healthy take-out food sections are on the increase. Salad and soup bars are standard offerings in supermarkets. There are more and more clever, healthful bottled condiments and sauces, such as pesto, chutney, tapenade, seasoned mayonnaise, and curry sauces, which can turn everyday ingredients into gourmet dishes—perfect for dressing up such basics as chicken or a fish fillet. And the range of healthy frozen entrées and side dishes you can choose from is broader than ever. Eating out is also an option. Once you become familiar with recovery foods, you will be able to spot them on menus and order dishes that best support your new regimen.

Introducing the Recovery Eating Goals

The nutrition program for recovery features seven goals, designed to help you make sure you're eating regular, healthy meals that will bolster your physical and emotional recovery. Goals 1, 2, and 3 ask you to make sure to eat the most nutritious foods, while Goals 4 and 5 tell you what to stay away from. Then Goals 6 and 7 ask you to fine-tune your food choices, focusing on quality of ingredients.

Goal 1: Eat three meals a day, including breakfast.

Goal 2: Have more fruits and vegetables.

Goal 3: Favor whole foods.

Goal 4: Stay away from junk foods.

Goal 5: Cut back on caffeine.

Goal 6: Make sure to eat a balance of healthy oils.

Goal 7: Choose more organic ingredients.

Of course, these goals are good advice for everyone, but in particular they are important for health for someone with a history of drinking. The person in recovery, though no longer imbibing, is still recuperating from the damage inflicted by alcohol and especially needs regular, wholesome meals, including breakfast. They have probably been eating poorly and therefore have a lot of nutritional catching up to do. The goals of cutting back on junk food and caffeine also have special meaning for former alcoholics. Many see abstinence as a green light to chow down on high-fat foods and sugary items as a reward for not drinking. Caffeine all too often becomes the next addiction, as former drinkers switch their allegiance to coffee or colas. Making the effort to eat the healthiest oils also deserves special attention, because certain oils can help offset such consequences of drinking as inflammatory disease and heart disease. Finally, eating more organic foods is strongly recommended to ease the burden of toxins on your liver, a vital organ that has long been under attack.

Keep in mind that we're painting with a big brush here—these are general targets, shifts in what you feed yourself every day. If you find yourself munching on something not particularly nourishing, some old standby sweet snack or a fast-food meal-on-the-run, just be sure to eat something healthy at your next meal, so you can get back on track. Say, for example, on Tuesday morning you find yourself grabbing a large coffee with double cream and a doughnut. The next day, try to have a smaller coffee with less cream, and a bran muffin. Or, if one day you have a hot dog with the works for lunch, the next day, order a tuna sandwich on multigrain bread with a side of coleslaw. And if one day you simply don't bother to eat and then binge on your favorite deep-fried take-out Chinese food for dinner, the next day, make sure to eat a normal breakfast, have perhaps soup for lunch, and make broiled fish for dinner. In the next chapter, you'll find menus for homemade meals and tips on eating out that will give you a way to put all the goals into practice.

Goal 1: Eat Three Meals a Day, Including Breakfast

While this may seem a very basic goal, it's well known that people who drink too much don't have a habit of eating three squares a day. In fact, in a large, nationwide study of health behaviors and alcohol consumption, conducted in 1998 at the University of Iowa, the more frequent and heavier the drinking, the greater the tendency to skip breakfast and to snack between meals. Heavy drinkers are also likely to eat haphazardly, skipping meals and ordering in pizza, calling this dinner. Pursuing this goal of having regular meals is a great first step, a way of sending yourself the message that, even though you may have been ignoring your health before as drinking took over your life, from now on you'll be taking care of yourself while you recover.

How do you fare when it comes to eating normal, regular meals? Even with abstinence, are you still following the eating routine of the alcoholic lifestyle? Yes, it takes some planning on your part to make sure you have nourishing food morning, noon, and night, but such effort will really pay off in terms of recovering your health. For one thing, regular meals help stabilize blood sugar. Simply eating more good food will also supply more nutrients, for greater energy and to help restore normal liver function. It's a good idea to start each day by spending a moment to consider what you'll eat at each meal, rather than figuring this out at the last minute when you're famished and likely to eat anything within reach. To help you with the meal planning, the next chapter gives twenty-one days' worth of menus, including breakfast, lunch, and dinner.

Breakfast: Required Eating

Breakfast gives your body something to run on from the get-go and can also set you on the right course for healthy eating throughout the day. You'll begin to develop a taste for real food rather than junk food, which may make it less likely you'll revert to bad eating habits from your drinking days. Conversely, several studies that examined health practices have confirmed that not eating breakfast is a risk factor for illness.

However, just having a bagel and coffee won't do. Sure, this sort of breakfast will give you a rush of energy—but will cause a drop an hour or so later, when you'll probably feel tired, foggy headed, and maybe even grouchy (no, not you!), a bit depressed or at least not as positive about the day as you felt when you were on your coffee high. Such blood sugar–dependent drama can be prevented by eating a decent breakfast, one that gives you some protein, some fat, and some starch. That's because a breakfast of all three basic major nutrients can supply you with a steady stream of energy over a period of time. When you eat starch, your body immediately breaks this down, giving you energy that lasts about an hour to an hour and a half. Next, protein, which takes longer to digest, kicks in after about two or two and a half hours; and finally, fat is converted to energy after three hours. So a balanced breakfast at 8:00 a.m. can carry you through to lunch. Both while in recovery and as you're holding to your commitment to abstinence, you need this kind of nutritional support. It helps to have sustained energy and the steady moods that go with this to break habits you've had for years. If you've become accustomed to a midmorning slump, your day can feel and look a whole lot better when you give your body the best fuel to assist your recovery!

There are lots of wholesome classic breakfast foods to choose from, starting with eggs, whole grains, and dairy products. Breakfast is also an easy way to include fruit and nuts in your diet. Get in the habit of making a good amount of fruit salad that will last you a couple of days, and top this with almonds or walnuts.

Goal 2: Have More Fruits and Vegetables

"Fruits & Veggies—More Matters" is the slogan developed by the Centers for Disease Control and Prevention and other health organizations to encourage Americans to eat more of these healing plant foods. As a whole, Americans have a fairly dismal record when it comes to produce intake. Only an estimated 10 to 20 percent of individuals consume even the minimum five servings a day, the recommendation based on the 2005 Dietary Guidelines for Americans. And people who drink too much aren't known for their ample intake of fruits and vegetables, either. And the target can be even higher. The updated guidelines also set a higher recommended goal of nine servings being ideal for most adults. Gulp! How much is that? Four and a half cups of fruits and vegetables. But don't panic. "Cup" doesn't refer to a vat of broccoli, just a standard 8-ounce measuring cup, what a single chopped-up stalk of broccoli would fill. Still, to make your daily quota, it's a good idea to get an early start and make sure you have some fruit with breakfast, or perhaps sautéed tomatoes or mushrooms with your eggs—like a first-class English breakfast! Then have some veggies as a salad, in soup, or in a sandwich for lunch, and include a vegetable side dish with dinner, plus some more fruit for dessert. Between meals, you might also snack on some vegetables, raw or cooked and dressed up with a sauce or dip.

If you're not already eating a lot of produce, just by following this guideline you'll be making a significant change in the way you eat and taking an important step in recovery. As mentioned in previous chapters, fruits and vegetables deserve to be a featured part of recovery meals. Abundant sources of fiber, vitamins, and minerals, they play a vital role in restoring the normal function of virtually all body systems, helping restore health to the bones, nerves, digestive tract, and liver. In addition, these fiber-rich foods can really fill you up, leaving less room for sugary and junk foods you may have noshed on in your drinking days. Eating fresh fruits and vegetables may also change your taste for food. Once you're accustomed to the flavor of "fresh" and the way your body responds to nutrient-packed ingredients, highly processed foods with overtones of chemical additives will begin to lose their appeal—I guarantee it! You won't have to promise yourself you'll eat better for your recovery; you'll want to.

Which Fruits and Vegetables Aid Recovery?

It's easy to give yourself a full range of nutrients by eating a variety of produce. Below you'll find lists of recovery fruits and vegetables likely to be found in the produce section of your supermarket or at farmers' markets, as well as at health food stores that carry fresh organic produce. Including all of these at one time or another in your meals will help your body repair. And as you continue to eat these superfoods, you can look forward to not just an absence of ailments but a new level of health compared with your drinking days that may go beyond your expectations in terms of energy and vitality.

Recovery Fruits:

Apples

Apricots

Bananas

Blackberries

Blueberries

Cantaloupe

Dates

Guava

Kiwis

Lemons

Mangoes

Oranges

Papayas

Peaches

Pears

Plums

Prunes

Raisins

Raspberries

Strawberries

Watermelon

Recovery Vegetables:

Artichokes

Asparagus

Avocadoes

Beets

Broccoli

Brussels sprouts

Cabbage (such as green, red, and napa)

Carrots

Cauliflower

Chicory

Corn

Cucumbers

Dark leafy greens (such as kale, collard, turnip, mustard, and beet greens)

Green beans

Lima beans

Mushrooms

Okra

Onions

Parsley

Peas

Romaine lettuce

Potatoes in their skins

Pumpkin

Spinach

Sweet peppers

Sweet potatoes

Tomatoes

Winter squash (such as hubbard, butternut, and acorn)

At the end of this chapter, you'll find food shopping lists that include these fruits and vegetables.

Goal 3: Favor Whole Foods

Because alcohol can undermine so many different aspects of body function, from the liver and digestive tract to the brain, the nutritional needs for repair are equally diverse. Consequently, for recovery you can't afford to eat refined and processed foods that are missing some of their vitamins, minerals, oils, fiber, and so forth. What you need is whole foods. "Whole" foods—foods that our grandparents would recognize—are foods that still retain all of their parts. "Whole" encompasses fruits and vegetables, which are better for you if you eat both the skin and pulp, and even the green tops when possible, for the extra fiber and nutrients these provide. Beans, nuts, and seeds are also whole foods.

"Whole" is also about grains. Take wheat, for example. A whole kernel of wheat contains over twenty vitamins and minerals, plus healthy oils and fiber. But when grain is refined, the germ and bran are removed, along with 97 percent of the fiber, 25 to 30 percent of the protein, and a significant percent of each of the nutrients. What's left is the large center section of

Buying Bread—Chewy, Not Squishy

Paying special attention to the kind of bread you eat is an important aspect of recovery eating because typical white bread can cause low blood sugar, a health issue for most alcoholics during their drinking days that can persist even with abstinence. What you want is bread that is chewy, a sign that it contains fiber and a good amount of whole grain, a source of many nutrients. A bread that is all processed flour, with no whole grains, can cause problems.

Flour is grain that has been pulverized and, consequently, during digestion, the grain is much more exposed to digestive enzymes. These rapidly break down the starch into sugars. Absorption speeds up as the small sugar molecules readily enter the system and blood sugar level quickly rises. Even fluffy whole wheat flour has this effect, although whole wheat is one step better than white bread. One kind of chewy bread you'll find in most markets is pumpernickel, made with whole rye kernels. Look for these small, heavy, rectangular loaves of thinly sliced bread displayed with other breads or near the deli section—since this pumpernickel goes well with such toppings as ham or smoked salmon.

When you go shopping for bread, what you want to look for on the label are the words "whole grain," and/or "kernels," which tell you that some of the grain in the product has been left intact and not milled into flour. You might see "wheat kernels," "oat kernels," "barley kernels," or the wheat kernel, the endosperm, which is mostly starch. Of course, white wheat flour is enriched, but with only five nutrients returned to it—the B vitamins thiamine, riboflavin, niacin, and folic acid, and the mineral iron. A cup of whole wheat flour contains 136 milligrams of magnesium, important for heart and bone health, whereas a cup of enriched white wheat flour contains only 28 milligrams. Zinc, part of the nutrient team that quenches free radicals and supports normal immune function, drops from 2.88 milligrams in whole wheat flour to 0.77 in refined wheat flour. And so forth.

Buying Bread—Chewy, Not Squishy *continued*

"whole wheat berry." "Cracked" wheat is another desirable term, which refers to the whole wheat berry broken into fragments. You also want to get some idea of how much whole grain is in the loaf. Check the ingredient list to find out. Remember, the list is given in order of the most abundant ingredients. You should also be able to easily see the whole grains in the actual loaf, embedded in a slice and possibly sprinkled all over the top.

Breads that are multigrain are also a good bet. Ideally, a loaf should include six or seven different grains, and be both whole grain and multigrain. At the same time, make sure to avoid breads that contain lots of different sweeteners, because of their empty calories and ability to raise blood sugar. Some breads contain high-fructose corn syrup, honey, molasses, and raisin juice concentrate, adding up to more sugar per slice than these separate listings suggest. You also want to make certain that any loaf you buy does not contain partially hydrogenated vegetable oil. Chapter 6 tells you how these oils undermine health. An excellent brand that meets all these qualifications is Ezekiel 4:9. Their sprouted, 100 percent whole-grain bread is flourless and has a low glycemic rating listed right on the label. It's also certified organic and a source of complete protein because the bread contains both grains and two legumes, lentils and soybeans.

A grain that is whole is called a *complex carbohydrate*. Complex carbs can decrease craving for alcohol, according to research conducted at St. Rita's Medical Center in Lima, Ohio. Nutritional therapy was added to a traditional rehabilitation program that was based on the Alcoholics Anonymous 12-step program. Some participants had only the traditional therapy, while others also followed a special diet that increased complex carbohydrate options. These latter patients reported less alcohol craving as well as higher nutrient intakes.

You don't have to go to a health food store to buy whole grains, although such places carry a greater variety than your local grocery probably does. But you should be able to find several kinds of whole grains in your supermarket. Look for the following:

Barley

Brown rice

Bulgur wheat

Cornmeal

Kasha (roasted buckwheat)

Rolled oats

Skipping Sugar

Sugar is also part of the "whole" story. Unless you are chewing on stalks of sugarcane, the sugar you normally eat is the refined kind. White sugar contains no vitamins, minerals, or fiber, just carbohydrates. The same goes for high-fructose corn syrup, which has poured into the American food supply in recent years, increasing by 135 percent in the last decade. Check labels and you'll find it in all sorts of baked goods and breakfast cereals, to name just a few of the food categories touched by this invasion. High-fructose corn syrup is worse for cholesterol levels than is saturated fat, increases bone loss, and contributes to fatty liver. To satisfy your sweet tooth, enjoy whole fruit instead.

Treasuring Whole Eggs

The elegant egg, with its fascinating shape and subtle color, deserves to be kept intact, with both the yolk and the white happily consumed. This perfectly balanced two-part food, with its mix of amino acids, is the gold standard for protein content. Nutritionists use it to measure the protein value of other foods. Because of this superior protein value, eggs make a great food choice for recovery, when body tissues need rebuilding. Each section of the egg also contains its own special vitamins and minerals, the ones in the yolk complementing and working together with those in the white. As for that cholesterol in the yolk, worry more about your intake of saturated fat when it comes to heart disease. You don't need to have a three-egg breakfast every day, but having an egg or two a couple times a week is fine. Think of eggs as the perfect fast food.

Goal 4: Stay away from Junk Foods

As much as eating for recovery is about the positive side of food, all the wonderful ingredients out there that you can enjoy, this way of eating doesn't cut junk food much slack. Eliminating highly processed, deep-fried, and fast food is absolutely necessary for true recovery, especially if you've been relying on these to keep you going up to now. You might think such advice is old hat, but not in this context. For someone with a history of drinking, staying away from junk food makes especially good sense—and studies back this up.

Eating lots of junk food increases cravings for alcohol. In a 1972 study published in the *American Journal of Clinical Nutrition*, animals fed a typical teenage "junk food" diet continuously increased their alcohol intake during the experiment. In contrast, another group eating a well-balanced control diet maintained a low level of alcohol intake. In another study, published in the *International Journal for Biosocial Research* in 1983, alcoholics who were hospitalized were fed either a hospital diet or a special diet that excluded junk foods. This regimen also eliminated caffeinated coffee, dairy products, and peanut butter (a potential allergen) but included fruit and wheat germ. Of those patients on the hospital diet, fewer than 38 percent were abstinent after six months, while 81 percent on the special diet remained sober.

Yes, junk foods can give you quick energy and, with their combination of salt, sugar, and fat, can be very appealing, but they don't truly nourish. This doesn't mean you should never eat at a fast-food outlet. Several of the chains are making a serious effort at including healthy salads and lean chicken sandwiches, as well as fruit and nut combos. Better to make a meal of these than to not eat at all. Just don't get lured into the burger and fries offerings while you're standing in line waiting to place your order.

Goal 5: Cut Back on Caffeine

For many recovering alcoholics, coffee drinking and other caffeine intake becomes woven into their new way of life. Coffee seems to be ever-present at support meetings and becomes the acceptable drink for socializing. Some people carry about and down colas as if this beverage were water. For many, the caffeine rush is seen as keeping them going, or preventing them from feeling grouchy. As one person in recovery said, "I no longer drink. Now I'm just on coffee." Yes, caffeine can keep you high just like alcohol— but it's dangerous, just like alcohol! It's very easy to get hooked on such "soft" beverages, despite the fact that they stress the adrenal glands, digestion, and the liver, all of which are in the process of healing.

Caffeine intake is also associated with alcohol cravings. In a study published in 1991 in the *Journal of the American Dietetic Association*, hospitalized patients with alcoholism who were given a special diet that excluded caffeine reported decreased cravings for alcohol four months after discharge. Their nutritional therapy also restricted sugar and increased complex carbohydrates. And in the animal study testing for the effects of junk food, cited under Goal 4, when caffeine and coffee were added to a junk food diet, alcohol intake increased.

Ideally, for full recovery of your health after abusing alcohol, you should eliminate all coffee, both caffeinated and decaffeinated, and any other sources of caffeine from your diet, especially if you are in the first stages of withdrawal. This includes sugary, caffeine-laced sodas, those energy drinks that deliver a major hit of caffeine. For example, a 16-ounce Rockstar delivers 160 mg of caffeine. Beverages made with caffeine-containing plants such as guarana and yerba maté also contain significant amounts of caffeine, as does nonherbal tea.

But if this request is the stopper, the one that gives you the excuse to also toss out the first four guidelines in this program—and maybe even this book—then a compromise is in order. Of course, this doesn't mean it's okay to walk around all day with your cherished coffee mug in your hand. But it's better to wash down that nourishing breakfast and all those servings of fruit and vegetables with a couple of swallows of coffee than to not follow this nutrition program at all. Stop drinking coffee and any other form of caffeinated beverages entirely if you can, but if you cannot, at least have a goal of cutting back to one to two cups of coffee per day or diminishing your daily intake of caffeinated soda or tea.

As your body adjusts to its changing chemistry, it needs to be sheltered from dietary stress. The problem with caffeine, when it comes to trying to restore your health after a history of drinking too much, is that it attacks the same body systems and functions that alcohol also interferes with. Take a look at these interactions:

Digestion. Coffee and tea, both regular and decaffeinated, increase the secretion of stomach acids, which in turn can lead to injury of the intestinal walls and a higher risk of ulcers, heartburn, and acid reflux. Coffee, with or without caffeine, can also have an unwanted laxative effect.

Liver detoxification. Caffeine further burdens an already stressed liver which now has the job of detoxifying and neutralizing this compound.

Adrenal glands. Caffeine increases the adrenal glands' output of stress hormones, including cortisol, which increases heart rate and blood pressure and puts the body in a state of emergency. Let's face it, all that high energy and mental clarity in a cup is why coffee is so beloved. But it can come with a big-time price—anxiety and adrenal exhaustion. Normally, the adrenal glands shut down when overly fatigued, but caffeine overrides this protective chemistry and keeps you going until you drop. Caffeine also stimulates appetite as part of this stress response, which can lead to food cravings—in particular, for sweets.

Blood sugar. Caffeine triggers a surge in blood sugar, but as little as two cups of coffee, or less in sensitive persons, can lead to an episode of low blood sugar, or hypoglycemia.

Brain chemistry. The brain produces a "feel-good" messenger called GABA (gamma-amino butyric acid) that can calm mood and the digestive tract, but caffeine blocks GABA's soothing effects.

Skeletal system. Osteoporosis is associated with alcoholism, and coffee may increase the risk of this disease. The acidity of coffee triggers the body to neutralize the acid by drawing alkaline minerals like calcium from the bones. Coffee and tea, caffeinated and decaffeinated, also stimulate the kidneys, further increasing mineral loss.

I've had to deal with caffeine dependence myself, but let's face it—constantly running your engine on this substance just doesn't work. A coffee or cola habit slows full recovery.

Tips for Cutting Back on Caffeine

Even though you may have now overcome your alcohol addiction, you may still be locked in caffeine addiction. Going cold turkey from caffeine can be very challenging, with withdrawal symptoms that include a major headache lasting for days, significant fatigue, and a drop in mood. Keep your goal the same but give yourself a break and cut back slowly, a doable approach that works just fine. Here are some tips for reducing your daily caffeine dose.

▸ First switch to regular tea, which has about half the caffeine as coffee. Then substitute herbal teas for some of the caffeinated kind.

How Big Is Your Coffee Cup?

A reasonable target for starting to cut back on caffeine intake is 200 mg or less per day. Higher doses in the range of 200-plus to 800 milligrams can produce nervousness and anxiety. If you are wondering how much caffeine you are giving yourself, consider what you call a "cup." Standard charts on caffeine content usually give the size of that cup as 6 fluid ounces. Good luck! That's not much coffee! A standard can of soup is about 15 ounces. That 6 ounces of coffee would fill less than half of that soup can! But when you go for take-out coffee, the "small" is likely to be 12 ounces; the medium, 16; and the large, 20. Now consider that the average amount of caffeine in 6 ounces of coffee, according to *Consumer Reports*, is 100 mg (based on a range of 70 mg to 215 mg). If the cup size is double or triple that? . . . you do the math.

Compared with coffee, 6 ounces of nondecaffeinated tea contains much less caffeine, 50 mg, but still a significant amount. Caffeinated soft drinks also deliver a dose of caffeine: a 12-ounce can of Coca-Cola contains 46 mg and Dr. Pepper, 41. Even decaf coffee contains a smidgeon of caffeine, 4 mg per 6 ounces. A word of caution: Although colas and some soft drinks contain less caffeine, they are not recommended for recovery. The caffeine can still add up and these beverages contain sweeteners and artificial ingredients. They are also very acidic, increasing the risk of osteoporosis as the body attempts to buffer the acidic effects of colas with minerals drawn from the bones.

▸ Swap some coffee for a caffeine-free coffee substitute. There are several new products on the market and my guess is you'll be totally surprised at how rich, pleasantly bitter, and satisfying these can be. These products are an inventive mix of ingredients such as roasted barley, chicory, figs, orange peel, rye, and toasted soy. Gourmet versions are scented with hazelnuts and Mexican chocolate. Look in the section Healthy Food Resources (pages 300–307) for brands. When you make filtered coffee, reduce the amount of ground coffee beans and add some coffee substitute instead. Try making some of your daily cups 100 percent the herbal kind.

▸ When you want an energy lift and sharper thinking, down a glass or two of water. Your problem may not be a lack of caffeine but dehydration and a lack of water. Caffeinated and decaffeinated coffee, as well as tea, are diuretics. To stay ahead of the fluid loss, for every one cup of coffee you drink, have two cups of water.

▸ When you want an energy and mood lift, start moving. Exercise is a proven cure.

▸ A more unusual but highly effective route is to work with an herbalist, such as a practitioner of traditional Chinese medicine, who can give you a bitter herb concoction. One of the great appeals of coffee is its special bitter taste. But when the body has had enough of this flavor, such as from bitter herbs—and I speak from experience—that coffee bitterness will be anything but appealing.

Goal 6: Make Sure to Eat a Balance of Healthy Oils

If you've been following the guidelines of this nutrition program for recovery, having a moderate amount of fat in your diet and limited saturated fat, thank yourself for sticking to one of the key components of recovery eating that can help protect your health. This is no small accomplishment, especially if you had been accustomed to eating lots of high-fat foods and snacks in your drinking days. But for optimal well-being, there's still room for improvement. You also need to eat the right combination of oils.

Which oils are best for health and how much of these is best? That depends on the kinds of polyunsaturated fats they contain. There are two kinds of polyunsaturated fats: the omega-3 essential fatty acids and the omega-6 essential fatty acids. (The 3 and the 6 refer to the different structures of a molecule of these oils.) Essential fatty acids are special fats, workhorses that make up a substantial part of cell walls and also have many vital biological functions. For instance, omega-3s reduce stress reactions and aid digestion.

When Essential Fatty Acids Are out of Balance

The typical American diet doesn't provide enough omega-3s and, in particular, people who abuse alcohol may not be consuming enough. According to data collected as part of the U.S. National Health and Nutrition Examination Survey and published in 2007 in *Alcoholism: Clinical and Experimental Research*, men who binge-drink have lower levels of omega-3s than do those who are not heavy drinkers. Such a deficiency can compromise brain function, which depends on having an adequate supply, and add to the damage to brain tissue that alcohol may already have caused. How the body uses fatty acids is also negatively affected by alcohol. Omega-3 fatty acids are also needed to offset the effect of the omega-6s. Omega-3s widen the arteries and thin the blood, whereas omega-6s narrow the arteries and thicken the blood. In addition, omega-3s are anti-inflammatory, versus omega-6s, which promote inflammation. The particular effects the omega-3s and omega-6s have on the system can be a factor in heart disease and inflammatory conditions such as hepatitis, diseases linked to alcoholism. The ratio of these two kinds of fats in your diet can affect your chances of recovering your health after a history of drinking.

The Ratio of Omega-6s and Omega-3s to Aim For

The best ratio of omega-6s to omega-3s for health, according to many experts, is in the range of 1:1 to 4:1, similar to the ratio in the American diet a hundred years ago. But in today's average diet, the ratio is closer to 10:1 and possibly as high as 20 to 25:1 in favor of omega-6s. The vegetable oils touted for good heart health in the 1980s are a major reason for this imbalance. Soybean, corn, and cottonseed oil are high in omega-6s and enter the food supply in abundance in the many food products made with these oils. Of course, you do need some omega-6s in your diet and for that reason safflower oil, a source of omega-6s, is one of the recommended oils for recovery. It makes the list because it's widely available in an unrefined version.

To maintain the right balance of omega-6s and omega-3s, here are some tips:

▸ Prepare more foods from scratch. Chapter 6 provides recipes for salad dressing, to help you avoid bottled dressings made with omega-6 oils.

Flaxseed Oil— Tender Care Required

Flaxseed oil is recommended for recovery because it's a source of essential omega-3 fatty acids. Because it is fragile and oxidizes easily, flaxseed oil must be protected from heat and light to prevent it from becoming rancid. In stores, it's kept under refrigeration and, at home, you need to do the same. Put your flaxseed oil in the fridge even before you've opened the container. And don't ever heat flaxseed oil when you're using it in cooking. Rather, add it to salad dressings and drizzle it on toast or over vegetables once they've been cooked.

▸ Add a splash of flaxseed oil to dishes, to boost their omega-3 content. Omega-3-rich flaxseed oil has a flavor that is somewhat nutty and a little like butter.

▸ Eat more fish, an abundant source of omega-3s. In chapter 6, you'll find lots of tasty recipes for cooking seafood.

▸ Snack on walnuts, the only common nut that contains omega-3s.

▸ Shop for grass-fed beef and eat some wild game, which feed on plants that contain omega-3s.

▸ Choose brands of eggs that announce on their cartons that the eggs inside supply omega-3s, produced by hens on an omega-3 diet.

Goal 7: Choose More Organic Ingredients

While this goal is important for everyone, it is especially key for anyone in recovery. Organic foods are those that are free of pesticides, growth

Staying Away from Trans Fats

Trans fats have no place in a recovery diet. These are man-made fats that cause malfunctions wherever they end up in your body. Trans fats have twice the negative effect on cholesterol as do saturated fats and also interfere with how the essential fatty acids function.

Trans fats form when an oil is partially hydrogenated; any product that contains partially hydrogenated oils contains trans fats. Common sources are commercial baked goods such as cookies, muffins, and crackers, and deep-fried food such as french fries and fried chicken, as well as many brands of margarines. You'll find the number of grams of trans fats per serving listed on the Nutrition Facts panel of food labels.

hormones, antibiotics, heavy metals, and chemical additives such as artificial flavors and preservatives. You don't want to be consuming these substances, especially while you're following a recovery regimen. Pesticides are designed to disrupt the cellular function of creatures that attack and damage plants and have the potential for doing the same in the human body. Any pesticides that the liver can't detoxify will accumulate and can do harm. At risk is the liver, GI tract, kidneys, and nervous system, areas of the body probably already weakened when there's been years of alcohol abuse. Pesticides can also be a factor in the development of various cancers. Studies have identified individual pesticides that lead to such problems. Now imagine the cumulative effect of consuming an assortment of pesticides, which is closer to reality for anyone eating a nonorganic diet. It is your liver's job to deal with these compounds once they're in your system. Limit your diet's toxic load and the liver can save its nutritional and biochemical resources for repair.

Going Organic—Where to Start

An easy way to start cutting back on your toxin intake is to begin buying organic dairy products such as milk and butter. Another effective tactic is

---

More Pesticides and More Organic Foods

According to the U.S. Department of Agriculture, in 1939, there were only 32 registered pesticide products, but by 1989 there were 22,000, containing one or another of 729 active ingredients. And in 1995, 1.25 billion pounds of pesticides were sold in the United States alone. Fortunately, the organic food business is also increasing at a dramatic rate. U.S. sales of organic food and beverages has grown from $1 billion per year in 1990 to over $15 billion in 2006. You have choices.

to purchase more organic produce. Of course, if you're like most people, as you're reading this you're already thinking "price." Organics can seem like a luxury because these items usually cost more than conventional foods do. But buying more organic foods is certainly cheaper than medical care, and there are ways to cut costs. Here are some tips to save you money.

▶ Shop at the big natural food emporiums that manage to lower price based on the volume of produce they sell.

▶ If price is a consideration, buy the weekly organic fruit and vegetable specials. Also, watch for reduced prices on introductory or house brands of organic foods at supermarkets.

▶ Check out the natural foods aisles at grocery stores and gourmet shops—but also look for organic items that have been integrated with conventional foods on the regular shelves. For instance, many supermarkets these days stock a few organic brands of pasta right alongside the processed brands.

▶ Swing by your local farmers' market and search out the producers who are raising their crops and animals organically or at least

Reducing Pesticides by Washing and Peeling

You can eliminate some pesticides by washing and peeling fruits and vegetables, but not entirely. And of course, along with the peel you'll be losing some nutrients, which tend to concentrate near the peel. One step you can take is to wash all produce in special rinse products made with natural ingredients such as lemon oil, grapefruit seed extract, or corn and coconut oil, designed to remove pesticides and waxes. Another strategy is to eat a variety of fruits and vegetables, to avoid a concentration of particular pesticides.

with minimal chemicals. Chat up the fellow selling the produce about how the product you are about to buy was grown or raised.

▶ Join an organic food co-op to beat the system and share in the savings. Go to www.localharvest.org to find a group in your area.

▶ Think of all that money you're saving by focusing on the recovery eating goals of not buying so many processed and prepared foods, as well as specialty coffee concoctions, and invest those dollars in organic foods instead.

▶ Check out the Web site for the Environmental Working Group, www.ewg.org. The EWG is a not-for-profit environmental research organization. They list forty-five fruits and vegetables, ranked from those with the most pesticides to the least. Here are the dozen conventionally grown foods with the greatest pesticide load, starting with the highest:

Peaches

Apples

Sweet bell peppers

Celery

Nectarines

Strawberries

Cherries

Lettuce

Grapes—imported

Pears

Spinach

Potatoes

If you can't always buy organic, at least make a point of eating produce with the lowest pesticide load. Here's a list, starting with the least pesticides:

Onions

Avocadoes

Pineapples

Mangoes

Asparagus

Kiwi

Bananas

Cabbage

Broccoli

Eggplant

You can download a Pesticides in Produce shopping guide when you go to the EWG Web site.

Shopping for Organic Meats and Poultry

Organic meats and poultry can be significantly more expensive than the conventionally raised versions and not always easy to find. But when you do decide to purchase some, here's what various labels on meats and poultry mean:

Organic meats. Animals are raised on organic feed that is free of synthetic pesticides, herbicides, artificial fertilizers, and genetically modified organisms (GMOs). They have not been injected with hormones to promote growth or given antibiotics to prevent the possible development of disease. And in the processing of the meat, no additives, sulfites, or synthetic coloring are added to improve texture, taste, color, or shelf life.

Organic poultry. Birds are fed only organic grains and given no antibiotics, artificial growth stimulants, or animal protein by-products. The grain is also GMO-free.

What Organic Product Labels Are Telling You

Cruise your supermarket aisles and you might discover such diverse organic products as frozen dinners, fruit juice, and ketchup. According to market research, 393 of 633 food and beverage categories now offer organic products. National standards for organic products finally became fully implemented and enforceable as of October 2002. Here are various organic product labeling terms and what they mean.

100% Organic
All organic ingredients
Any processing aids used must be organic
No nonorganic ingredients used
USDA seal allowed
Must list certification agent
Example of ingredients listing: 100% organic cereal

Organic
At least 95% organic ingredients by weight, excluding water and salt
Remaining 5% can be nonorganic allowed ingredients (e.g., vitamins, citric acid, baking powder)
All agricultural ingredients must be organic unless not available

Residue-free meats. These meats are from animals that may have received preventative antibiotics or hormones to promote growth at some point in their lives. However, at the time of slaughter, the meat contained no traces of these.

Free-range chickens and turkeys. This only means that the animals were raised in outdoor pens, not inside buildings.

What Organic Product Labels Are Telling You *continued*

USDA seal allowed
Must list certification agent
Example of ingredients listing: organic cereal

Made with Organic Ingredients
At least 70% organic ingredients
Remaining 30% can be nonorganic allowed ingredients (e.g., vitamins, citric acid, baking powder) or nonorganic agricultural ingredients
USDA seal prohibited
Must list certification agent
Example of ingredients listing: cereal made with organic oats, raisins, and dates

Products with Less Than 70% Organic Ingredients
Any level of organic ingredients
No restrictions on remaining ingredients
No certification claims can be made
USDA seal prohibited
Only mention organic in ingredient listing
Example of ingredients listing: organic oats, organic raisins

Food Allergy/Intolerance and Alcoholism

As you begin to put into practice the goals of recovery eating, another step to take is to become more aware of food allergies and intolerances. Identifying food sensitivities can be a vitally important aspect of recovery. Food allergies (which involve the creation of antibodies by the immune system) and intolerances (which do not) can worsen ailments associated with alcoholism. If a person is sensitive to a food, eating it can make him or her ill. Health problems associated with food allergy or intolerance are extremely varied and can affect many of the same body functions also affected by drinking. See the sidebar on "Testing for Food Allergies" on page 89 for a list of symptoms. You may never have even considered you had a food intolerance or allergy, but clinicians who treat alcoholism have found that a good number of people who abuse alcohol do. In one study, published in 1987 in the *International Journal for Biosocial Research*, among one hundred alcoholic patients, 73 percent were found to have food allergies. The most common allergenic foods were wheat (58 percent), milk (50 percent), beef (22 percent), corn (22 percent), eggs (14 percent), and peanuts (14 percent).

A food that a person is sensitive to can also become addictive. If you're sensitive to wheat, for instance, you may not be able to stay away from wheat for a few days without really craving some. What's happening is that the food is triggering the production of endorphins, feel-good, morphine-like compounds, as the body works out a way to adapt to the allergen. When you stop eating that food, no endorphins are produced and withdrawal occurs, along with other symptoms such as fatigue, brain fog, fluid retention, headache, poor digestion, low blood sugar, anxiety, depression, and even anger and abusiveness. What stops the symptoms is more of the offending food, and now an addiction has begun.

If the food in question is, for instance, eggs, the addiction problem is limited to eggs and foods that contain eggs, but when the food is also an ingredient in some alcoholic beverage, then the addiction can extend to that drink. For example, a person sensitive to corn may crave bourbon, which is

Testing for Food Allergies

Patch and RAST (blood) allergy tests disclose true allergies but miss food intolerances that do not engage the immune system. Another standard test used by physicians and dietitians to identify food allergy or intolerance is the elimination diet. First, the patient eliminates certain foods from the diet for one to three weeks. Typically, most or all of the commonly eaten foods are avoided and, if health improves, the foods are reintroduced one at a time, while monitoring the patient for symptoms. Some doctors also require the patient to fast before starting this process. The patient usually feels worse for a few days and then notably much better on day six or seven.

You can begin by doing some of your own allergen sleuthing. If you think you may be sensitive to an ingredient, keep a food and symptoms diary, to connect the dots of whether exposure to a substance causes any of these common reactions either immediately or within the next day or two:

▶ Heart palpitations; difficulty breathing or swallowing; or swelling of the lips, tongue, or throat
▶ Diarrhea or other digestive disturbances
▶ Mouth numbness or tingling, dryness, blisters, or a sense of "fuzziness"
▶ Nasal congestion, coughing or hoarseness, or sneezing
▶ Eye redness or swelling of eyelids
▶ Headache or dizziness, pressure in your ears
▶ Hives, eczema, or other skin eruptions, or itching
▶ Depression, anxiety, fatigue, or confusion

If you identify a possible dietary culprit, does eliminating the food alleviate the symptom(s)? Discuss with your physician whether and how you should take measures to continue to avoid the food. In most cases, substitutions can be made to permit you to continue to enjoy your favorite dishes.

principally made from corn. Someone who does not tolerate potatoes may be addicted to vodka made from potatoes. Much research on these associations was conducted starting in the mid-1940s by a pioneer in environmen-

Making Food Substitutions

Making substitutions for foods that you are sensitive to is a huge subject in itself, since various suspect ingredients show up in so many food products. But here are some tips for starters:

▶ Replace dairy products with products made with soy. Mainstream grocers as well as health food stores sell soymilk, soy ice cream, and soy cheeses—even soy "whipped cream." Also give rice milk and rice ice cream a try. Almond milk is another option (if nuts are not also a problem). And look for vegan products, which by definition do not contain even trace amounts of dairy ingredients. Vegetarian or lactose-free items may still contain casein, a milk protein that can spark the allergy.

▶ If eggs produce a reaction, consult vegan cookbooks to learn how to cook and bake without eggs, including substituting ground flaxseed beaten with water in baked goods. Replace standard grains like wheat and corn with rice and more unusual grains such as millet and quinoa. Gluten-free cookbooks offer a range of recipes that omit wheat and, often, corn products.

▶ If you find you're allergic to corn, also eliminate wheat, which is closely related from an allergy viewpoint.

▶ Read labels very carefully. Some versions of products may include common allergens; for example, "real" forms of mayonnaise are supposed to be dairy-free and corn-free, but Kraft olive oil mayonnaise contains lactic acid, which could cause problems for people with a lactose intolerance, and Hellmann's olive oil mayonnaise contains cornstarch, a no-no for people who cannot have corn.

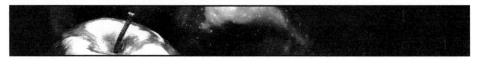

tal medicine, the clinical ecologist Theron G. Randolph, MD. Working with patients, he monitored their reactions to various alcohol products and traced these back to related food allergies. Patients reported having hangover symptoms even from eating just the allergenic foods. To treat their particular alcohol addiction, he had them avoid both the drink and the food, as eating the food helps perpetuate the craving. Symptoms such as fatigue and headache subsided and even their craving for alcohol disappeared.

Randolph discovered that identifying the food origins of an addiction to alcohol could be quite complicated, since various substances may sneak into alcohol products during manufacture. For instance, some rums are made purely from sugarcane whereas others may contain a small amount of grape brandy. All-malt whisky is made of roasted barley or malt, while blended Scotch whiskey contains some whiskey made with corn. Drinks may also contain rye, yeast, and other possible allergens. The only way to know if you have an actual sensitivity to any of these ingredients is to undergo extensive food allergy testing, as well as observing your symptoms when you consume such foods. Foods that you crave and consume very regularly are likely suspects.

Heading into the Kitchen

Cooking can be even easier when your kitchen is organized and well stocked. Setting up your kitchen for cooking saves lots of time and effort later. This section tells you how to check to be sure you're ready.

Outfitting Your Kitchen with the Right Equipment and Foods

The following lists of cooking equipment and foods will set you up for cooking the meals and recipes in this book. Right now you may not think you need a colander, but at the moment you want to drain the pasta, you will want a colander. Better to be prepared than have to improvise. It's also nice to be able to simply reach on your shelf for a can of tomatoes when you need one. Here's a chance to feel in control of your world!

Clearing the Decks

Take an inventory of what you have sitting on your kitchen shelves and tucked away in the refrigerator. Anything not really healthy goes, such as pork sausage and juices that contain high-fructose corn syrup. Throw out all the sugary stuff, like breakfast cereals that taste as sweet as candy. The same goes for any products with ingredient lists that contain lots of added chemical compounds meant to flavor, color, and preserve the product, substances that tax your liver.

You will also want to toss food that's old, like stale crackers, a forgotten box of oatmeal, beans you bought last year, and frozen leftovers of a certain age. Check expiration dates on all packaged goods. Give items a sniff. Stale grains, especially whole grains like brown rice that have been around for a while, smell musty. Also remove any sources of alcohol that might tempt you to drink and even any drinking paraphernalia and barware, the sight of which might trigger a craving. Give your body and mind all the support you can.

The following gives you some good rule-of-thumb timelines for various foods:

▸ Cornmeal and oats stay fresh in the pantry for up to 6 months.
▸ Whole grains, stored in a tightly sealed container in the refrigerator, are good for 3 months.
▸ Beans keep in the pantry for 1 year but are best used within 6 months.
▸ Cooking oils can be kept at room temperature for up to 6 months.
▸ Nut oils, such as walnut oil, require refrigeration and stay fresh for up to 3 months.
▸ Frozen leftovers are best in flavor and texture eaten within 1 month.
▸ Herbs and spices lose flavor after 1 year. Throw out any suspect ones and buy fresh. You'll notice the difference in how your food tastes!

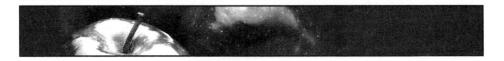

If you don't cook or truly have only the very basics in your kitchen, these lists may look overwhelming. You don't have to go out and buy all this stuff at once, to start feeding yourself healthy foods. But glance over the following and begin to assemble some proper equipment, offered in the spirit of efficiency and to make your cooking easier.

BASIC KITCHEN GEAR

Pots and pans:

2 skillets: 8-inch and 12-inch

1 ridged grill pan

4 pots: 2- or 3-cup, 1 to $1^{1}/_{2}$ quarts, 4 quarts, 8 quarts, plus lids

Covered casserole, 6 to 8 quarts

9 x 13-inch metal roasting pan

12-cup muffin tin

Baking sheet for french "fries"

3 mixing bowls: small, medium, and large

Appliances:

Toaster

Blender, for shakes and soups

Food processor, for easy chopping and combining

Slow-cooker or Crock Pot

Utensils:

2 cutting boards, wood or plastic, 1 for most produce and 1 for
  meat, onion, and garlic

Paring, chef, and bread knives

Long-handled spoons: one wooden since it doesn't heat up like metal, one large stainless-steel spoon for transferring and serving food, one slotted spoon to drain liquids from food

Ladle

Wide metal spatula

Measurers: a 2-cup glass or plastic cup for liquids, a set of $1/4$ cup to 1 cup dry measures, a set of measuring spoons

Colander

U-shaped vegetable peeler

Metal rack for roasting meat

Instant-read thermometer, the most accurate way to determine doneness of meats

Whisk, for quick mixing without using a food processor

Salad spinner, a fun way to dry all those greens you'll be eating

Collapsible metal steamer, for cooking vegetables while retaining their nutrients

Bamboo skewers, 6- or 9-inch, for stove-top grilling

Becoming an Expert Food Shopper

To make sure you're buying the best foods for recovery, label reading is a required skill.

You especially need to check for fat content, the amount of saturated fat in the product, the sugar content, and the number of artificial ingredients. You'll find this information on the Nutrition Facts panel and also in the ingredients list. But before you read further, grab a can of soup or a box of something and take a look at the label so you can follow along with the explanation below.

Fat figures. As you see, the Nutrition Facts panel tells you the percentage of fat and the percentage of saturated fat in the food. Since the recovery diet targets keeping total fat to 30 percent of calories and minimizing saturated fat, you don't want to eat a product that gives you, for instance, 50 percent of your daily allotment of fat or 40 percent of your saturated fat quota in just one serving.

Also make sure the Nutrition Facts panel states that the product you're buying contains no trans fats. Another way to avoid trans fats is to never buy a product made with partially hydrogenated vegetable oil.

Sugar ranking. Check the ingredients list for the sugar content. The closer an ingredient is to the beginning of the list, the more there is in the product. When a muffin or a cereal has sugar placed first or near the top of the list, you know you'll be getting a lot of these empty calorie carbohydrates when you eat this food. Another sign is when the ingredients list contains several different kinds of sugars. See the sidebar on page 96 for the names of these. Check for sweeteners even in foods that you don't think of as sweet, for instance, ketchup and salad dressings. Sugar is added to an enormous range of products. That's why, according to the USDA, the average American eats about 64 pounds of added sugars each year. These include table sugar, corn syrup, honey, and high-fructose corn syrup.

Sneaky serving sizes. While you're checking for percentage of fat and carbs on the Nutrition Facts panel of a product, also take a look at the serving size that these percentages refer to. You'll find serving size stated near the top of the panel. I'm warning you, you could be in for a big surprise! Sometimes this amount is much smaller than how much you're likely to eat, unless you stop at two crackers, an ounce of cheese, or half a cup of ice cream. If you eat double or triple these amounts, then double or triple the stated percentage of fat in a serving to know how much you'll actually be eating.

Outstanding Recovery Foods

So many different foods can help you in recovery that you may begin to wonder what to eat first. To help you decide, here are those especially beneficial foods that, again and again, show up as recommended ingredients. Make a photocopy of this list and keep it in your wallet or in the glove

---

Aliases for Sugar

Be aware of the many names for sugar. Often several sweeteners are listed and, if combined, could earn sugar a place at the head of a product's ingredients list.

Corn syrup
Corn sweeteners
Dextrin
Dextrose
Evaporated cane juice
Fructose
Fruit juice concentrate
High-fructose corn syrup
Honey
Invert sugar
Molasses
Malt
White grape juice

compartment of your car. Add other healthy foods as you begin to follow the many eating tips and cook the recipes in this book, and you'll soon create your own useful personal shopping list for recovery.

Your Recovery Pantry

Make it easy to eat healthy recovery foods by making sure you keep some on hand. Create a recovery foods pantry. You might start with a reserve of rolled oats and some whole-grain breakfast cereal, to have handy some of the recommended grains. Then add some buckwheat pancake mix or tabbouleh mix and some whole-grain bread crumbs. Have a store of canned and bottled beans and bags of dried legumes. Bring home such healthy canned goods as tomatoes, pureed pumpkin, salmon, chopped clams, chunk light tuna, and fat-free, low-sodium chicken stock. Also sample the new boxed soups and stocks that have especially fresh flavor. And buy some all-natural peanut butter.

Treat yourself to bottled sauces, syrups, condiments, and dressing that add flavor and help you quickly put together tasty meals. Shop for spaghetti sauce, pure maple syrup, prepared mustard, salsa, all-fruit spreads, and low-fat dressings such as vinaigrette and Caesar. It's best to make your own salad dressing with top-quality oils using one of the recipes in chapter 6, but better to top a salad with one of the healthier commercial kinds than eat no salad at all. A word of caution: These products can contain added sweeteners, preservatives, and artificial flavors, so be sure to read labels. When available, make sure to buy brands that use a minimum of additives, such as Newman's Own and Amy's.

Also give yourself a well-stocked freezer. Make sure it holds frozen chicken parts, chicken or turkey patties, frozen shrimp, and flash-frozen fish fillets as well as frozen lima beans and frozen soybeans (edamame). You'll also be glad to reach in and find bags of frozen strawberries, blueberries, and mango.

To make it easier for you, I've compiled this list of Recovery Pantry Staples. Most all of them are called for to prepare one or another of the

The Top Recovery Foods

VEGETABLES:
- [ ] sweet red peppers
- [ ] beets
- [ ] spinach
- [ ] asparagus
- [ ] artichokes
- [ ] avocadoes
- [ ] cauliflower
- [ ] cabbage
- [ ] Brussels sprouts
- [ ] broccoli
- [ ] chicory
- [ ] kale
- [ ] sweet potatoes
- [ ] tomatoes
- [ ] okra
- [ ] onions
- [ ] cucumbers
- [ ] parsley
- [ ] winter squash

FRUIT:
- [ ] bananas
- [ ] pears
- [ ] apples
- [ ] papayas
- [ ] mangoes
- [ ] strawberries
- [ ] blueberries
- [ ] watermelons
- [ ] cantaloupes
- [ ] oranges
- [ ] lemons

GRAINS:
- [ ] oats
- [ ] brown rice
- [ ] barley
- [ ] whole-grain and rye breads

LEGUMES:
- [ ] all beans
- [ ] lentils
- [ ] peas

SEAFOOD:
- [ ] salmon
- [ ] tuna
- [ ] herring
- [ ] sardines
- [ ] shrimp

POULTRY:
- [ ] turkey
- [ ] chicken (and eggs)

DAIRY:
- [ ] organic yogurt
- [ ] milk
- [ ] butter

NUTS:
- [ ] walnuts
- [ ] almonds
- [ ] Brazil nuts
- [ ] peanuts

SEEDS:
- [ ] flaxseeds
- [ ] sunflower seeds

DRIED FRUIT:
- [ ] raisins
- [ ] cranberries

SEASONINGS AND HERBS:
- [ ] fresh garlic
- [ ] caraway seeds
- [ ] dill seeds
- [ ] rosemary
- [ ] cardamom
- [ ] turmeric
- [ ] cinnamon
- [ ] ginger

OILS:
- [ ] extra-virgin olive oil
- [ ] unrefined safflower oil
- [ ] flaxseed oil
- [ ] butter substitutes

BEVERAGES:
- [ ] filtered tap water
- [ ] mineral water
- [ ] herbal teas
- [ ] coffee substitutes

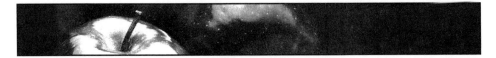

meals in the twenty-one recovery menus that follow in chapter 5. Some are basic foods, like canned tomatoes and raisins, but I've also included certain gourmet and exotic ingredients, such as capers and curry sauce. If alcohol has dampened your taste buds, you can look forward to new pleasures with these intriguing condiments and sauces.

You needn't buy all these foods at once but do purchase at least a half dozen or more to get your pantry started. You'll also be building your pantry when you shop for the ingredients to prepare the meals in chapter 5's menus. A time saver is to do one big shopping trip once a week, planning ahead what you'll be eating in the next several days. Select three or four of the menus, check their recipes and the ingredients called for, and stock your kitchen with these. You'll have what you need when it's time to cook, and what you don't use of the nonperishables can go into your pantry or fridge.

RECOVERY PANTRY STAPLES

Soups: canned low-sodium chicken broth and lentil soup; bottled beet borscht; boxed soups such as squash, tomato, and sweet red pepper; boxed chicken and vegetable broth

Canned vegetables: tomatoes, pureed pumpkin

Cereals: rolled oats, whole-grain breakfast cereal

Grains: refrigerated tubes of polenta, whole-grain couscous, whole-grain bread crumbs, brown basmati rice, tabbouleh mix, buckwheat pancake mix, pasta

Legumes: canned black beans, dried lentils, frozen peas, lima beans, frozen soybeans (edamame)

Fish: canned chunk light tuna, salmon, and chopped clams; frozen shrimp; and flash-frozen fillets

Poultry: frozen chicken parts; frozen chicken or turkey burgers; and turkey sausage

Nuts, seeds, and dried fruit: almond butter, peanut butter, plus the nuts, seeds, and dried fruit in the Top Recovery Foods list (page 98)

Herbs and spices: thyme, mixed Italian herbs, bay leaves, summer savory, cumin, chile powder, curry powder, allspice, plus the herbs and spices in the Top Recovery Foods list

Vinegars: balsamic vinegar, rice vinegar

Condiments and flavorings: prepared mustard, salsa, mayonnaise, capers, tapenade, all-fruit spreads, mango chutney, toasted sesame oil, vanilla powder

Sauces, syrups, and bottled dressings: spaghetti sauce, pesto, soy sauce, pure maple syrup, salad dressings such as vinaigrette and Italian, Chinese hoisin sauce, Asian peanut sauce, curry sauce

5 THE DAILY EATING PLAN

Menus for Recovery

IT'S YOUR TURN NOW to put all this advice on what to eat for recovery into practice—starting with the recovery meals in this chapter. As a nutritionist, I've seen first hand the ill effects of alcoholism as well as the healing properties of food. The following twenty-one menus give you a way to immediately take advantage of these benefits. They feature the supernutritious recovery foods that can support you in restoring your health.

These menus, for breakfast, lunch, and dinner, feature easy-to-prepare comfort foods like chili, pork chops, and pancakes. You don't have to turn your life upside down to comply with this meal plan. The menus work even for hectic days. You also don't have to be a whiz at cooking: Many of the meals only require combining a few ingredients, such as canned pumpkin and chicken broth to make "squash" soup. If you know how to boil water and turn on the stove or broiler, you'll do just fine.

Keep in mind that the eating plan presented in this book is not a demanding regimen but a workable method of transition from how you eat now to a healthier approach to food that you can stick with for life. You'll find it allows some wiggle room, nutritionally speaking. While eating whole foods is a target goal, recipes include some white flour and sugar here and there, and although the meals include lots of fruits and vegetables, you'll also need to snack on some to eat the recommended daily amount—which takes care of any worries you may have that you can't eat between-meal snacks. Using these meals as a foundation, you'll find yourself better nourished, with more energy, steadier moods, and clearer thinking; you will also be less susceptible to minor ailments. These menus set you on the road to your goal of total recovery.

The way the meals are arranged is designed to give you, over a period of a day or two, approximately 20 percent protein, 30 percent fat, and 50 percent carbohydrate, the profile of the recovery diet. A dinner consisting of this proportion of nutrients might start with bean soup, a small salad with vinaigrette, and move on to a main course of chicken, a serving of potato and a vegetable, with a baked apple for dessert. Of course, specific dishes will be higher in one or another of these basic nutrients but, on average, the menus fit this scheme. Foods that supply healthy oils are favored over sources of saturated fat. There is also no calorie counting per se. Eating wholesome foods in moderate quantity, and no longer taking in extra calories from junk food and alcohol, should be sufficient to prevent weight gain.

Why Twenty-one Menus?

Giving you twenty-one days' worth of eating was done by design. Researchers found that in three weeks to a month, a person can reprogram his or her tastes and habitual food choices. In this short amount of time, you're likely to be eating more fruits and vegetables without much thinking about it, while junk foods will start to lose their appeal. Stay with these menus for two to three months and you'll truly be launched into a new era of eating and full recovery.

Tips for Following This Plan

One way to begin eating for recovery is to simply start with Menu 1 and continue to eat your way through consecutively to Menu 21. In fact, going in order makes good sense since, in some cases, what you cook on one day becomes part of a meal on the next. That said, you can also vary the schedule. For example, you might repeat a day's menus every once in a while if you have lots of leftovers that need to be eaten. It's also fine to prepare the suggested lunch menu for dinner or vice versa, or skip a day of eating your own food and have all your meals in restaurants. (You'll find tips on recovery foods to order when eating out at the end of this chapter.) Lots of combinations work, with one major exception: Don't make a habit of eating just a single day's menu over and over, even if the ingredients in the dishes are very healthy. Only a variety of foods can deliver the full range of nutrients you need. March through these menus or meander. Either way is fine, as long as you keep going. The point is to begin to let your body experience what it feels like to be fed wholesome, nourishing foods over an extended period of time.

Of course, I do understand that as you begin to change your eating style, on some days a less-than-ideal meal might just sneak in there—and that's okay. The process of changing how you eat will likely have its ebb and flow. If you haven't been accustomed to regular meals, even having a daily breakfast might be a challenge. When resistance hits, I wholeheartedly encourage you to stick to your resolve to eat better. And remember, there's no need to beat yourself up for making a side trip into the world of fries and colas. Use it as a test to see how your energy and spirits fare after a couple of meals like this, compared with how your new way of eating lets you feel. Healthier foods will win out, I promise. Look back after three months of consuming wholesome foods and you'll be glad you started truly nourishing yourself. Just make sure to keep your eating habits going overall in the right direction and you'll have good reason to congratulate yourself.

Your Recovery Menu

As mentioned above, the breakfast, lunch, and dinner of each day's menu have been carefully thought through so that the combination of foods is appetizing and the combination of meals also gives you the right mix of carbohydrates, fats, and proteins. The menus also work together in terms of themes, with the next day's offerings a refreshing change from what came before. These menus are designed to give you reasons for buying healthy ingredients, resulting in a kitchen that is well stocked with recovery foods. Enjoy!

PHASE ONE MENUS:

Menu 1:
Breakfast: Rolled oats with milk and banana
Lunch: Greek salad with feta cheese and stuffed grape leaves
Dinner: Store-bought roasted chicken with whole-grain couscous, squash, and salad with oranges and walnuts

Menu 2:
Breakfast: Fruit salad with yogurt and sunflower seeds
Lunch: Sliced chicken sandwich with chutney on whole-grain bread
Dinner: Canned turkey chili topped with avocado and salsa

Menu 3:
Breakfast: Baked apple with almond butter toast
Lunch: Lentil soup and Greek salad pita pocket
Dinner: Frozen healthy entrée and dinner salad

Menu 4:
Breakfast: Ready-made polenta with prosciutto and melon
Lunch: Onion soup and grilled cheese sandwich
Dinner: Salad bar stir-fry with brown rice and egg drop soup

Menu 5:
Breakfast: Mexican-style eggs with corn tortillas
Lunch: Ham sandwich with fresh pineapple and cottage cheese
Dinner: Salmon sandwich with a cup of fresh asparagus soup

Menu 6:
Breakfast: Cold cereal and fruit
Lunch: Mediterranean sampler: tapenade toast, prosciutto and melon, mixed greens salad with chicory
Dinner: Pasta primavera with pesto

Menu 7:
Breakfast: Healthy breakfast shake
Lunch: Chicken hot dog with three-bean salad
Dinner: Roasted turkey breast with baked sweet potatoes, peas, and pearl onions

Menu 8:
Breakfast: Oatmeal with vegetarian breakfast patties
Lunch: Creamed herring on whole-grain rye bread with Danish apple and beet salad
Dinner: Turkey and avocado sandwich with apricot-almond crisp

Menu 9:
Breakfast: Spinach-egg scramble with rye toast
Lunch: Pizza and arugula salad
Dinner: Garlic shrimp with black beans, brown rice, and sautéed bananas

Menu 10:
Breakfast: Pan-fried tomatoes with baked beans on toast
Lunch: Healthy frozen entrée
Dinner: Indonesian chicken saté with peanut sauce and cucumber salad

Menu 11:
Breakfast: Yogurt-berry sundae
Lunch: Gazpacho and Southwest chicken burger
Dinner: Angel hair pasta with clam sauce and Italian-style garlic spinach

Menu 12:
Breakfast: Buckwheat pancakes with homemade fruit sauce
Lunch: Meat loaf sandwich
Dinner: Grilled salmon on a bed of warm corn and lima bean salad

Menu 13:
Breakfast: Diner breakfast: poached eggs and home fries
Lunch: Curried "squash" soup with peanut butter and banana sandwich
Dinner: Turkey sausage, polenta, and kale

Menu 14:
Breakfast: Dinner leftovers
Lunch: Sautéed sweet red pepper salad and goat cheese
Dinner: Pork chops with sautéed onion and apple, plus sweet-and-sour red cabbage and egg noodles

Menu 15:
Breakfast: Whole-grain breakfast cereal
Lunch: Salad bar minestrone soup
Dinner: Fish and fries with deli coleslaw

Menu 16:
Breakfast: Meal in a muffin
Lunch: Beet soup and egg salad sandwich
Dinner: Steak salad with sweet red peppers

Menu 17:
Breakfast: Breakfast in a muffin with Canadian bacon
Lunch: Chicken salad with avocado and papaya
Dinner: Turkish meatballs with traditional side dishes

Menu 18:
Breakfast: Smoked salmon cream cheese on whole-grain bread
Lunch: Tabbouleh salad with Turkish dinner side dishes
Dinner: Grilled halibut with tapenade, served with boiled potatoes and Greek-style green beans

Menu 19:
Breakfast: Oatmeal with poached gingered pears
Lunch: Salade Niçoise with pesto baguette
Dinner: Frozen chicken enchilada with pinto beans and Mexican rice

Menu 20:
Breakfast: Waffle Danish
Lunch: Herb frittata
Dinner: Seafood supper

Menu 21:
Breakfast: Herb frittata with yogurt cheese
Lunch: Crab cakes
Dinner: Curry in a hurry

Your Recovery Meals

These twenty-one menus give you suggestions for the core of the meal, such as the main dish at breakfast, the salad at lunch, and the entrée at dinner. What's missing, of course, are all the snacks, desserts, and beverages that would round out these daily menus. But don't worry. You'll find suggestions for snacks at the end of the menus, on pages 156–157. And chapter 6 includes entire sections on desserts and beverages.

Vegetarians Welcome!

In recovery eating, there's a place at the table for vegetarians, too. Eating meat and poultry is not required to make use of nutrition to repair the body damaged by alcohol. In fact, the great majority of ingredients recommended for recovery are plant foods, anyway. Fruits, vegetables, nuts, seeds, grains, and legumes are what supply the many vitamins, minerals, phytonutrients, and fiber necessary for recovery. Animal foods also offer important vitamins and minerals but, as any vegetarian knows, plant foods can supply equivalent sources. In addition, the seven goals of this eating plan can be applied to a vegetarian diet as well as to one that is not. Making sure to have three meals a day or go organic has nothing to do with eating meat. And because eating for recovery limits saturated fat, for the health of the liver and heart, a vegetarian diet can even be superior to one that is nonvegetarian, since plant foods in general are lower in this kind of fat compared with animal foods.

The eating suggestions and recipes in this book offer lots of vegetarian options. You'll find that many of the suggested meals can be prepared in a vegetarian version. Menu 4's dinner, salad bar stir-fry with brown rice and egg drop soup, can be made with chicken or not, and the Turkish dinner on Menu 17, with its vegetable and chickpea side dishes, is still nourishing without the meatballs. Also look through the lunch suggestions for vegetarian dishes, such as lentil soup and herb frittata. Other vegetarian meals can be assembled by combining nonmeat dishes whose recipes appear in chapter 6: Legumes and grains go together to give you quality protein. Add a vegetable dish and you have a meal.

Even if you are not a vegetarian, you might want to consider substituting fish for a meat dish in some of the menus. Seafood gives you special essential fatty acids, EPA and DHA, which are vital for health. (Strict vegetarians can take EPA or DEH capsules of fish oil. Vegans can take oils derived from algae.) Also try eating no animal products one or two days a week. You now have good reason to consume more vegetables, nuts, and legumes—and a chance to experience how energizing and satisfying a vegetarian meal can be.

The menus listed below provide simple steps for assembly, as well as the "recovery benefits" of each day's meals. Detailed recipes are listed in chapter 6; every recipe has the exact page reference, so it's easy to locate.

Menu 1

Breakfast: Rolled oats with milk and banana

You're off to a good start with oats for breakfast. Oats are one of the few common grains that usually come to market in a whole, unrefined form. But all oat cereals are not equally good for you. Oat groats, the whole kernels, take a long time to cook and are very healthy and very, very chewy; and oatmeal, which is also the groats but flattened with huge rollers, is fine. But instant oatmeal, whose flakes have been chopped into itty-bitty pieces, can rapidly raise blood sugar, since these digest quickly. Instant oatmeal products also contain added sweeteners that cause blood sugar to rise even faster. Stay away from instant oats, to speed recovery.

Oatmeal: Follow instructions on the package to prepare one serving of oatmeal. Top with ¹/₂ cup 2% milk and ¹/₂ sliced banana.

Lunch: Greek salad with feta and stuffed grape leaves

This salad, an easy go-together dish, makes for a satisfying meal, thanks to its variety of highly complementary ingredients: feta for protein and olive oil for long-lasting energy. You won't leave the table hungry when you have had this salad. See page 220 for the recipe.

Dinner: Store-bought roasted chicken with whole-grain couscous, squash, and salad with oranges and walnuts

The ubiquitous supermarket cooked chicken is a solid source of protein that can be the handy basis of meals over several days, an incentive to make sure you feed yourself something nourishing. Whole-grain couscous, which is actually semolina pasta cut into small bits, is a classic quick and easy food, and supplies fiber. The squash provides vitamin A and fiber; the salad contains vitamin C, potassium, and healthy omega-3 oils.

This dinner requires several pots but little cooking. The chicken is "buy and slice." If you have high blood pressure and need to restrict your sodium intake, buy a no-salt-added chicken. The couscous cooks in a bowl just by

Lunch on the Job

If you happen to work in an area where you have a choice of quality restaurants, and you also have cash on hand for lunch and enough time to eat out, then giving yourself a healthy midday meal won't be a problem. Just consult the suggestions at the end of this chapter on what to order in various kinds of restaurants, and you can't go wrong. Quality restaurants and ethnic eateries offer lots of suitable-for-recovery dishes on their menus.

But if you're like the great majority of folks, and your lunch options are limited to fast-food joints and the local deli, then you owe it to yourself for recovery to brown-bag it, at least most days of the workweek. Consult the lunch suggestions of the recovery menus for ideas about sandwiches, soups, and salads that you can make ahead and cart to work. Bring Menu 2's sliced chicken sandwich made with chutney or Menu 13's curried "squash" soup to heat in the office microwave oven, and be prepared to receive envious glances and be asked for a taste.

You also have options if you manage to only bring part of a lunch or your workplace doesn't have a microwave oven. For instance, for Menu 3, brown-bag the Greek salad pita pocket and buy some soup if you can't bring lentil soup from home. For Menu 11, bring the gazpacho but, instead of the chicken patty sandwich, buy an egg salad sandwich. And Menu 9 is designed to start with purchased pizza but you bring the quality arugula salad. Of course, some of the suggested lunches require more cooking, soaking up hot water. The squash heats up quickly in a pot and you can just toss and serve the salad.

Store-bought cooked chicken: Slice and serve.

Couscous, preferably whole grain: Follow the package instructions. To flavor the couscous, add a pinch of cinnamon and a teaspoon of raisins

---

Lunch on the Job *continued*

such as Menu 18's tabbouleh salad and crab cakes in Menu 21. Plan these for weekends and days off.

Of course, nutritious brown-bag lunches such as these take some planning. To make a sandwich quickly in the morning, you might want to assemble the ingredients the night before, to have them in easy reach. If you'll be bringing a salad to lunch, such as the apple and beet salad in Menu 8, this keeps well and can be made the day before. You can also borrow some cooking time from the evening before and cook a lunch item that doesn't take much attendance, such as the salad bar minestrone soup of Menu 15, while you're cooking or eating dinner. Or have some of the soup for dinner and bring along some of the remaining soup in a Thermos jar to work.

Making this extra effort to plan a healthy lunch can really pay off in terms of recovery. You won't have to take a break from the wonderful effort you're making at other meals, to stick with your new way of eating— and you'll reap some immediate benefits. You'll feel a lot better the second half of your working day than if you had a fast-food burger and fries. You'll have more energy, and you'll be better able to think clearly and be more effective on the job. You won't conk out at 3:00 p.m. because you had deep-fried, sweet-and-sour shrimp for lunch, with all its fat and sugar. You probably won't even need as much coffee to stay awake. These kinds of improvements can help you get your life back on track, as you will be able to literally feel the program working its beneficial effects.

per serving to the water before bringing to a boil. Then pour the flavored hot water over the grain. (A gourmet option for raisins are the huge, plump, tawny beauties made with red grapes. Look for the Pavitch brand.)

Squash: Heat frozen pureed orange winter squash, such as Hubbard, in a small amount of water in a covered pot. (If cooking fresh squash, steam or bake in a 400°F oven for 1 hour.)

Orange and Walnut Salad: See page 220 for the recipe.

———————————— ☙ ————————————

Recovery benefits of Menu 1 foods

▸ Oats support healthy liver function by supplying soluble fiber, which promotes the flow of bile and detoxification.

▸ Fresh, raw vegetables in the Greek salad give you more nutrients than do the same foods cooked.

▸ Chicken, especially the dark meat, supplies easily absorbed zinc, a nutrient that may be depleted, since the body requires zinc to detoxify alcohol. Chicken is also a source of iron, another deficiency associated with drinking too much.

▸ Orange-colored squash is an abundant source of vitamin A, commonly deficient in alcoholics. To replenish reserves, the plant form of vitamin A, beta-carotene, which this vegetable supplies, is preferred to animal sources of true vitamin A, which at high doses can be toxic.

▸ Walnuts give you anti-inflammatory oils that help prevent heart disease, and the dressing made with walnut oil gives you a bonus dose.

Menu 2

Breakfast: Fruit salad with yogurt and sunflower seeds

This salad is an easy way to make certain you eat enough fruits for the day, one of the goals of this nutrition program for recovery. The antioxidants in colorful fruits protect the liver from damage by free radicals. Yogurt can help repair the GI tract. And sunflower seeds are powerful little packets of nutrition that supply nutrients good for the bones and circulatory system. These include the minerals potassium, iron, zinc, calcium, magnesium, manganese, and copper, plus vitamin B_6 and niacin. Make sure to buy your sunflower seeds from a store with good product turnover, which helps ensure they are fresh.

As for the fruits in the salad, you can always use just a single kind, like delectable white nectarines from a farmers' market in the heart of summer, or treat yourself to mixed fruit salad. The prep requires taking a bit of time as you wash, trim and slice all the fruits, but enjoying the result is an effortless luxury. You're worth it! Start with the following suggestions and then invent your own favorite combinations.

▸ Blueberries, peaches, pears

▸ Cantaloupe, strawberries, green grapes

▸ Mangoes, pineapple, bananas

To prepare: Wash the fruits. Peel those with thick skins and rinds, such as mango and cantaloupe, but keep the thin skins on apples and the like to give yourself some extra fiber. Cut the fruits into pieces and discard the seeds or pits. Top with low-fat yogurt and sunflower seeds.

Lunch: Sliced chicken sandwich with chutney on whole-grain bread

Having some leftover roasted chicken on hand may make it more likely that you'll not skip lunch. Enjoy it the second time around spiked with sweet-savory Indian mango chutney, available bottled in most grocery stores. Compared with white bread, the whole-grain bread gives you extra magnesium and zinc, minerals you need for your heart and immune system.

To prepare, slice the chicken and make a sandwich with a smear of chutney, the chicken, and some lettuce.

Dinner: Canned turkey chili topped with avocado and salsa

The beans in chili are a low-fat source of protein. Topped with avocado, this dinner also delivers folic acid and heart-healthy oils, and the onion in the salsa dampens chronic inflammation. Corn tortillas, unlike flour tortillas, are an excellent source of calcium. Get a head start on tomorrow's breakfast by baking an apple as you cook dinner.

Turkey chili: Read labels when shopping for canned chili, to check the fat content. Turkey chili and vegetarian chili are usually good bets. Heat according to the directions on the can. Spoon the chili into a bowl and top with sliced or chopped avocado and store-bought or homemade fresh salsa (see page 262 for the recipe). (To store unused avocado, wrap it in plastic wrap, with the pit intact, and refrigerate. The pit will keep it from turning brown.)

Corn tortillas: An easy way to "steam" tortillas is to heat them in a microwave oven. Stack three on a plate, sprinkling a few drops of water on each before laying down the next, and heat for 30 seconds. Or, if you prefer your tortillas crunchy, a nice contrast to the smoothness of chili, make your own chips. See page 262 for the recipe.

Baked apple: Bake while you dine, to prepare ahead for tomorrow's breakfast. See page 275 for the recipe.

─────────────────── ❧ ───────────────────

Recovery benefits of Menu 2 foods

▸ Strawberries, like other berries, help maintain steady levels of blood sugar, thanks to their high fiber content that gives them a low glycemic index.

▸ Sunflower seeds are one of the best sources of vitamin E, a powerful antioxidant, as well as essential fatty acids and an array of other nutrients.

▸ Beans in chili supply soluble fiber, which lowers cholesterol. They also provide calcium and magnesium, which strengthen bones, lessening the risk of osteoporosis associated with heavy drinking.

▸ Avocados supply folic acid, a B vitamin often missing in the diet of someone who drinks too much.

▸ Onions lower the risk of high blood pressure and stroke, two ailments particularly associated with binge drinking. Eating onions raw, as in this salsa, is most beneficial.

───

Menu 3

Breakfast: Baked apple with almond butter toast

Fruits such as baked apples take well to the additional richness of nuts, hence the almond butter toast in this handy breakfast. You'll find almond butter in natural foods stores, along with other nut butters such as cashew and macadamia, all worth sampling for their unique flavors. Almonds are high in heart-healthy monounsaturated fats. If you can't find almond butter, peanut butter—a quality brand with no added sugars or partially hydrogenated oils—is a good substitute.

Baked Apples with Cranberry Chutney: See page 275 for the recipe.

Almond butter toast: Spread 2 tablespoons of almond butter on a toasted slice of whole-grain bread.

Lunch: Lentil soup and Greek salad pita pocket

Lentil soup: If you're not accustomed to eating beans, having lentils is a workable first step. Lentils are relatively easy to digest, and they are easy to find in various canned soups available in most grocery stores. You can add to the nutrition and enhance the flavor of canned lentil soup with a squeeze of lemon juice, a source of vitamin C; some chopped fresh parsley, which is food for digestion; and/or a handful of fresh spinach leaves, to fight cancer.

Greek salad pita pocket: Start with the remaining Greek Salad ingredients of Menu 1—feta, tomato, lettuce, scallions, and stuffed grape leaves. Cut each into pieces small enough for easy eating in a pocket of whole wheat pita bread. Toss together in a bowl and fill the pita pocket with this mixture. Drizzle with bottled or homemade Greek salad dressing (see page 268 for the recipe).

Dinner: Frozen healthy entrée and dinner salad

Many frozen entrées available today are light years ahead of the TV dinner of the past, in terms of variety of dishes and the quality of ingredients. Hungry for a gourmet meal, such as a strip of salmon wrapped around a creamy, herb-scented filling, or some Thai noodles, or perhaps an Indian curry? You can find it frozen. And many products are made with organic ingredients. See page 303 for some recommended quality brands, and check the freezer cases of natural foods stores.

More stores are also carrying precooked meats, so you can quickly and easily create a dinner featuring pot roast, rack of lamb, or *carne asada* (a Mexican dish made with grilled pork). Add side dishes such as seasoned brown rice, green vegetables, and/or root vegetables that have been conveniently baked in the oven (see pages 199 and 200 for recipes for baked carrots and beets). You can also start with a precooked meat and build a dish from there. Begin with the pot roast and turn it into beef stew with the addition of potatoes, carrots, and onions.

Dinner salad: Complement your frozen entrée with something fresh, such as a nice dinner salad on the side. For instance, prepare a mix of baby lettuce greens, walnuts, and slices of pear in a honey-mustard dressing; or romaine, store-bought croutons, Parmesan cheese, and garlic vinaigrette. Use bottled dressings or make your own (see pages 268–272). Or make yourself some nourishing Carrot Slaw (see page 221 for the recipe).

Recovery benefits of Menu 3 foods

▶ Apples contain insoluble fiber, which can prevent toxins that interfere with the absorption of food and nutrients from forming in the digestive tract.

▶ Almond butter beats the kind of butter that comes from cows, when it comes to saturated fat. Nut butters get their richness from healthy monounsaturated fats.

▶ Lentils supply thiamine, which may be deficient in someone with a history of drinking; alcohol causes this vitamin to be poorly absorbed.

▶ A nice dinner salad on the side, which only requires a little fixing, is required eating to boost your daily intake of vegetables, especially when you've saved some cooking time by having a ready-made entrée as the main course.

▶ Raisins in the carrot salad supply inulin, a compound that stimulates the kidneys to clear toxins from the system.

Menu 4

Breakfast: Ready-made polenta with prosciutto and melon

Look for tubes of polenta in the grains section of your market. This specialty food from northern Italy makes a great breakfast food—it's similar to our own Southern cornmeal mush. Continue the Italian twist by enjoying it with prosciutto, a salt-cured ham, available in gourmet and Italian markets and some supermarkets. It's usually sold in transparently thin slices. Salty prosciutto makes a great flavor combination with a juicy, sweet fruit like cantaloupe. See page 180 for the Breakfast Polenta recipe.

Or eat your polenta as you would pancakes, prepared as in the Breakfast Polenta recipe but omitting the prosciutto and melon, instead topped with a drizzle (not a torrent!) of real maple syrup and an egg over easy.

Lunch: Onion soup and grilled cheese sandwich

French onion soup served in a restaurant typically comes topped with toast and melting cheese. Making this soup from scratch takes some effort, so here's a shortcut to the same combinations of flavors: easy onion soup coupled with a separate grilled cheese sandwich—a quick and satisfying lunch.

Onion soup: Start with canned onion soup, and add a pinch of dried thyme, a sprig of fresh parsley, and some freshly ground pepper. Follow the label instructions for heating.

Grilled Cheese Sandwich: See page 258 for the recipe.

Dinner: Salad bar stir-fry with brown rice and egg drop soup

That salad bar in your local supermarket can turn into dinner when you know how to stir-fry—a Chinese cooking technique that involves cooking vegetables in oil over high heat while briskly and almost constantly stirring and tossing the ingredients. Bring home from the salad bar an assortment of raw vegetables and some pieces of cooked chicken. You then add the Chinese flavorings: hoisin sauce (a reddish-brown sweet and spicy condiment) and toasted sesame oil. This oil isn't one of the featured oils for recovery eating because it's refined, but it deserves a place in the following recipe for its delectable, rich flavor. You'll find both hoisin sauce and toasted sesame oil in the ethnic foods section of the supermarket. Also toss in some peanuts. Easy-to-make egg drop soup gives you an appetizing first course.

Salad Bar Stir-Fry: See page 240 for the recipe.

Brown rice: Look for precooked brown rice packaged in a cooking bag that only requires dropping in hot water and heating for a few minutes, or start from scratch and cook super-flavorful and aromatic brown basmati rice for 40 to 50 minutes, using 2 cups of liquid to 1 cup of rice.

Egg Drop Soup: See page 213 for the recipe.

Recovery benefits of Menu 4 foods

▶ Corn is a source of fiber, thiamine, and vitamin C, and is a grain that tastes great at breakfast, served with such savory additions as the prosciutto in this meal.

▶ Onions contain sulfur compounds that go to work helping the liver inactivate potentially harmful substances, such as excess medications and undesired hormones.

▶ Brown rice, unlike refined white rice, delivers a big dose of magnesium, which is good for the bones. Bonus points for this whole grain!

▶ The veggies that are the basis of this stir-fry dinner prove how easy it is to eat cupfuls, a goal of recovery eating, when you've cooked them quickly and dressed them up with a tasty sauce.

▶ Peanuts have earned their place in heart-healthy diets, according to large and highly trusted studies. They're packed with a wide assortment of vitamins and minerals, giving good value for calories.

Menu 5

Breakfast: Mexican-style eggs with corn tortillas

One of the easiest ways to make sure you're giving yourself a nourishing meal is to keep a carton of eggs on hand in your refrigerator. Eggs are an excellent source of protein, inexpensive, quick to cook, and also good for dinner. Mexican Poached Eggs is based on a classic Mexican recipe in which eggs are poached in a chile-tomato broth. But in this case, instead of starting with broiled tomatoes blended with fresh chiles and onions, you can simply open a can of stewed tomatoes and use them for the sauce. See page 169 for the recipe. Enjoy with corn tortillas, a source of calcium.

Lunch: Ham sandwich with fresh pineapple and cottage cheese

Instead of a deli ham and cheese sandwich, brown bag this lunch, which gives you the same combo of foods but you control the quality of the ingredients. Select a reduced-fat ham and low-fat cottage cheese to cut back on your intake of fat, a burden for the liver. And make the sandwich with whole-grain bread and a smear of prepared mustard for a gourmet touch. Then add to your day's intake of fruit with a serving of fresh pineapple. Average portions would be $1/2$ cup of cottage cheese and 1 cup of fruit, but have more if you're hungry.

Dinner: Salmon sandwich with a cup of fresh asparagus soup

Soup and a sandwich can make a filling, healthy supper. This particular version features healthy fats—fish oils in the salmon—coupled with a rich yet fat-free soup. It's okay to have some dairy products and their saturated fat but, in this day's menu, you're already having cheese at lunch, so it's a good idea to cut back on saturated fat for dinner. This dairy-free soup is one way to do that. The thickener is rolled oats, which provide soluble fiber. If you have some cooked potatoes on hand, you can also substitute those, using the same amount as for the oats. This soup is made with asparagus, but you can use the recipe as a formula and substitute another vegetable instead. Try broccoli or cauliflower.

Savory Salmon Sandwich: See page 259 for the recipe.

"Cream" of Asparagus Soup: See page 214 for the recipe.

Recovery benefits of Meal 5 foods

▶ Tomatoes contain lycopene, a potent antioxidant that's been shown to lower the risk of esophageal, oral, and breast cancer, all associated with abusing alcohol.

▶ Cottage cheese, as part of a light lunch, supplies sufficient protein and some fat, to help maintain steady blood sugar levels until your next meal or snack.

▶ Canned salmon is a rich source of calcium when you include some of the softened fish bones in your sandwich, a tasty way to prevent osteoporosis.

▶ Asparagus is a top source of glutathione, a powerful antioxidant that also helps send fat-soluble toxins out of the system.

Menu 6

Cold cereal and fruit

The cereal aisle of your grocery store most likely has lots to choose from, but you'll need to read labels to make sure you select one that's best for recovery eating. Most commercially produced cereals are high in sugar (yes, even many that are labeled "natural"), so when you read the label, keep an eye out for all the names under which sugar may appear as an ingredient (see page 96 for a list of these). Remember, the closer to the first of the list an ingredient is, the greater the quantity. Products that contain whole grains, such as Kashi 7 Whole Grain Puffs, will give you some fiber, important for clearing toxins from the digestive tract. This cereal is also sugar-free, as is Grape-Nuts, another good bet.

Cereal fruit: Bananas are a handy cereal fruit, as are berries, since they don't require much preparation. Look for luxurious raspberries, strawberries, and blueberries. Sold frozen by the bagful, these berries are usually much less expensive than their fresh counterpart and can be a welcome change from apples and pears in winter, when fruit selection is limited.

Lunch: Mediterranean sampler: tapenade toast, prosciutto and melon, mixed greens salad with chicory

Sometimes having just hors d'oeuvres can make a satisfying meal, like going to a cocktail party but without the cocktails! This buffet, comprised of tapas classics of Mediterranean eating, is easy to put together.

Tapenade toast: Spread prepared olive tapenade (look for it in the condiment section of your supermarket) on toasted slices of French baguette.

Prosciutto and melon: Slice some cantaloupe or honeydew melon and wrap a piece of prosciutto around each piece. These days, you can find this gourmet version of ham in supermarkets as well as at Italian specialty stores.

Mixed greens salad with chicory: Start with a few leaves of chicory, a lettuce sold in upscale markets, and combine them with a handy bag of mixed lettuces already washed and chopped (rinse and pat dry all the greens before serving). Or combine the pleasantly bitter flavor of chicory with a source of sweet, such as sliced oranges. Dress with a basic vinaigrette. This is especially good with the tapenade toast and goat cheese.

Other side dish options:

▸ Canned Italian butter beans, which you can marinate in oil and vinegar

▸ Prepared caponata (a Sicilian condiment of eggplant, onions, tomatoes, anchovies, olives, pine nuts, capers, and vinegar)

▸ Goat cheese products flavored with garlic and herbs

Dinner: Pasta primavera with pesto

One of the goals of recovery eating is to include more vegetables in your meals, to supply you with all the many healing nutrients they contain. Pasta primavera features an abundance of sweet red bell peppers, broccoli, and cherry tomatoes—all featured foods for recovery. See page 183 for the recipe.

Note: This recipe calls for regular pasta made with refined wheat flour, to appeal to most people's tastes and to lure you into making this dish, which is loaded with vegetables. But to meet another goal of the nutrition program—to eat more whole foods—at least once, when you're making this dish, try upgrading the pasta to one of the many whole-grain varieties. New products have a lighter taste than you might expect. Also, for variety, try the milder-flavored pasta made with spelt, a type of wheat, or brown rice pasta. Spinach pasta is another healthy and tasty choice.

Recovery benefits of Menu 6 foods

▸ Blueberries are a recovery food for the brain, helping it to grow new neurons and improve the communication between them.

▸ Whole grains are associated with healthier levels of cholesterol, insulin, and blood sugar, according to a recent Danish study.

▸ Chicory, a salad green with curly, somewhat bitter leaves, has recognized medicinal properties. Chicory promotes the discharge of bile from the gallbladder, thereby assisting in cleansing the system of toxins that leave the body via this route.

▸ Hors d'oeuvres for lunch offer the option of nibbling, which may be more appealing than eating a full meal. Someone in the early stages of alcohol withdrawal may have problems digesting large amounts of food at one time.

▸ Garlic combats chronic inflammation, and raw garlic, the kind in this pesto sauce, is more potent than when cooked.

Menu 7

Breakfast: Healthy breakfast shake

Eating for recovery can include drinking for recovery—when the beverage is a healthy breakfast shake. These drinks are ideal, when you don't have the time or desire to cook. They also can deliver enough energy to last until lunch and give you a head start on meeting your vitamin and mineral quota for the day, if you make them with the right ingredients.

▸ Make your shake with whole fruit rather than fruit juice, to increase your fiber intake and help steady blood sugar.

▸ Give yourself some protein, with dairy and/or soy ingredients.

▸ Include a source of fat, like low-fat yogurt, rather than using only nonfat ingredients, for lasting energy.

Foundation ingredients for protein:

Low-fat yogurt

2% milk

Soy milk

Silken tofu

Peanut butter

Almond butter

Whole fruit for sweetening:

Bananas

Strawberries

Blueberries

Mangoes

Exotic flavorings:

Cinnamon

Cumin

Cardamom

Fresh mint

Fresh grated ginger

Healthy add-ins:

Protein powder

Freshly ground flaxseeds

Wheat germ

Liquid vitamin/mineral supplements

To start making breakfast shakes, use the Basic Breakfast Shake recipe on page 166 and follow it for a sense of quantities of ingredients. But go ahead and let your taste be your guide and have some fun concocting your own specialties.

Lunch: Chicken hot dog with three-bean salad

Chicken hot dog: Make this lunch with an uncured chicken hot dog and you'll avoid the nitrites in the usual kind of frankfurter. Nitrites combine with amines, a by-product of the way your body digests protein, and form potent carcinogens called *nitrosamines*. Since alcohol abuse is associated with a higher risk of several kinds of cancer, including those of the GI tract, you want to avoid these compounds. Applegate Farms and Organic Prairie offer both chicken and turkey uncured hot dogs that are also organic. Hot dogs made with chicken or turkey are also lower in saturated fat than are those made with beef.

The three-bean salad: Prepared mixed bean salad, which usually consists of red (kidney) beans, garbanzo beans, and green beans, is a no-fuss way to start to include more beans in your diet. But be sure to drain the beans before serving, because they are bottled in a sugary dressing. You can also simply make your own, without the sugar; see page 194 for the recipe.

Dinner: Roasted turkey breast with baked sweet potatoes, peas, and pearl onions

In an era when snacking and making do with fast food passes for "eating," having a square meal built around turkey can be a rarity, something that happens on Thanksgiving. But you can enjoy a substantial holiday-style meal whenever you wish, when you prepare the easy dishes in this dinner menu. Even if you're cooking for only yourself, you can enjoy roasted turkey without generating tons of leftovers, now that markets sell just the leg or breast. And wait until you savor a sandwich the next day, made with turkey you've cooked. What a difference from the rubbery deli version.

Baked Turkey Breast: See page 247 for the recipe.

Baked Sweet Potatoes: See page 211 for the recipe.

Peas and Pearl Onions: You'll find this a standard vegetable combination in the freezer section of your market. Follow the heating instructions on the package.

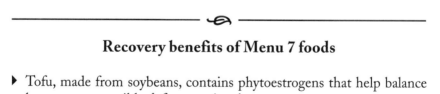

Recovery benefits of Menu 7 foods

▶ Tofu, made from soybeans, contains phytoestrogens that help balance hormones, a possible defense against breast cancer.

▶ Chickpeas, a common component of three-bean salad, provide folic acid, which also plays a role in preventing cancer.

▶ Turkey breast is lower in saturated fat than red meat and provides B vitamins that help manage stress and reduce fatigue.

▶ Mangoes offer a generous mix of antioxidants—beta-carotene, vitamin C, and vitamin E—plus a good amount of fiber.

▶ Sweet potatoes (also known familiarly as yams) are an abundant source of the plant form of vitamin A, beta-carotene, as might be guessed from their tawny orange color. These potatoes have a lower glycemic index than do regular white potatoes, making them the preferred choice for controlling blood sugar when you're hungry for spuds.

Menu 8

Breakfast: Oatmeal with vegetarian breakfast patties

If you are a vegetarian, you probably have already tasted sausage patties made with soy. If you're not vegetarian, the very idea of soy anything may be a giant turn-off. But trust me, give it a try. Forget about how fledgling products may have tasted way back when. These days, many kinds of soy sausage really deliver on appearance, texture, and savory flavor. Trader Joe's Breakfast Patties, for example, are a winner. One serving is 2 to 4 ounces. These products are usually very low in fat and contain no saturated fat at all, but give you some morning protein to fuel your early hours. They are also a good choice for breakfast if, later in the day, you plan to treat yourself to something creamy, such as the creamed herring that is the lunch offering in this day's menu. To prepare soy sausage, just follow the package instructions.

Oatmeal: Follow the instructions on the package to prepare one serving of oatmeal. Top with ¹/₂ cup of 2% milk.

Lunch: Creamed herring on whole-grain rye bread with Danish apple and beet salad

You'll notice that fish shows up on many of these menus, and for good reason. The oils in seafood prevent heart attacks and help the brain mend. Fish such as salmon and herring are staple foods in Scandinavia for both breakfast and lunch, displayed on open-faced sandwiches. In the deli section of your supermarket, you'll find small jars of herring. Creamed herring makes for a luscious lunch, especially on chewy slices of whole-grain rye bread, which is full of fiber. Just arrange a portion of herring on the bread; if the jar contains greater than one portion, refrigerate the leftover fish to enjoy another day. To round out this lunch and add to your fruit and vegetable intake for the day, serve with apple-beet salad.

Danish Apple-Beet Salad: See page 221 for the recipe.

Dinner: Turkey and avocado sandwich with apricot-almond crisp

One of the best sandwich combinations imaginable is sliced turkey breast and avocado, two delicate flavors and textures that merge into one delectable morsel. Complete this sandwich with a smear of cranberry sauce. Remember, you don't have to wait until Thanksgiving to relish these native American berries. And finish your supper with a generous scoop of fruit crisp. The recipe for the crisp is lengthier than most others in this book, but mixing the ingredients and assembling the dish is easy.

Turkey and Avocado Sandwich: See page 260 for the recipe.

Apricot-Almond Crisp: See page 276 for the recipe.

———————————— ᔆ ————————————

Recovery benefits of Menu 8 foods

▸ Beets contain a compound called betaine that, according to animal studies, protects against fatty infiltration of the liver caused by alcohol. It's thought that betaine does this by generating the formation of another compound, SAM (S-adenoslymethionine), which plays a significant role in maintaining the integrity of the liver.

▸ Herring replenishes reserves of vitamin E, which may be depleted.

▸ Dill contains limonene, which supports liver function by readying toxins for elimination.

▸ Pears are a good source of fiber, supporting healthy digestive function.

▸ Soy sausage is a good choice for recovery because it spares you the saturated fat of the usual pork sausage.

▸ Cranberries contain a red pigment shown in lab tests to prevent the oxidation of LDL "bad" cholesterol. Oxidation is what makes it more likely to lead to blood clots.

Menu 9

Breakfast: Spinach-egg scramble with rye toast

This breakfast helps ensure you are giving yourself a serving of green leafy vegetables, a source of magnesium that is good for the heart. The trick to having this dish come out right is to make sure you squeeze out all the juice from the cooked spinach, or your eggs will be watery. Spinach liquid also contains oxalic acid that binds with minerals, reducing the amount of the nutrients that your body has a chance to absorb. Enjoy this dish with rye toast and you'll be increasing the variety of grains in your diet.

Spinach-Egg Scramble: See page 170 for the recipe.

Lunch: Pizza and arugula salad

Pizza is a fast food that has some redeeming qualities. The standard kind comes with tomato sauce, which contains cancer-fighting phytonutrients. Add sweet peppers and mushrooms and you'll give yourself a serving of vegetables. Ask for extra garlic and your pizza will dampen inflammation. Enjoy a slice for lunch along with some salad made with arugula, an Italian salad green with a peppery, mustard flavor.

Pizza: Check your local natural foods store for frozen versions made with organic ingredients and whole-grain flour, such as Amy's pizza.

Arugula salad: You'll find this sold in bunches; prewashed and cut, in bags; as well as part of gourmet lettuce mixtures. Toss with vinaigrette and serve alongside the pizza or, gourmet style, mounded on top.

Dinner: Garlic shrimp with black beans, brown rice, and sautéed bananas

This dinner is inspired by Cuban cooking. Your body will benefit, thanks to the protein in both the shrimp and beans, two low-fat sources.

Garlic Shrimp: See page 231 for the recipe.

Black beans: Add a crushed clove of garlic, plus 1 tablespoon of olive oil, to a 15-ounce can of beans and cook them, covered, over medium heat in a small pot until heated, about 5 minutes. Cooked this way, the beans develop a depth of flavor with little effort on your part.

Brown rice: Follow the instructions on the package for cooking the rice, but use chicken broth as the liquid rather than water, for a richer taste. Try brown basmati rice, which is more aromatic than standard brown rice.

Sautéed Bananas: See page 265 for the recipe.

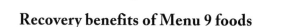

Recovery benefits of Menu 9 foods

▶ Spinach contains the two most important antioxidants in the body, glutathione and alpha-lipoic acid. With age, your body produces less of these, making spinach a tasty way to supplement them.

▶ Arugula, with its pleasantly bitterish flavor, may help you wean yourself off coffee, substituting for the satisfyingly bitter taste of java. It's worth a try!

▶ Bananas are a source of melatonin, a sleep-inducing and stress-relieving hormone, while they also sooth the stomach and help treat and prevent stomach ulcers.

▶ Rye is a source of vitamin E, which can become depleted with heavy drinking because the system uses this nutrient as an antioxidant as liver cells are damaged and the oxidation of fats increases.

▶ Egg yolks contain a nutrient called choline, which promotes the flow of bile and helps move fats in and out of the liver, counteracting fatty liver disease commonly associated with drinking.

Menu 10

Breakfast: Pan-fried tomatoes with baked beans on toast

Tomatoes contain lycopenes, phytonutrients that may help prevent cancers of the stomach and esophagus, a risk for some people who drink too much. Lycopene is better absorbed from cooked tomatoes and when eaten with some fat, as in this breakfast.

Pan-Fried Tomatoes: See page 207 for the recipe.

Baked beans on toast: This time-honored English breakfast is a warming way to begin a rainy day. Buy beans that have a savory sauce rather than one so sweet that the beans would qualify as a dessert. To prepare, simply pour the canned beans into a pot and heat them while you cook the tomatoes and make whole wheat toast. Spoon the beans over the toast.

Lunch: Healthy frozen entrée

Use this lunch as an opportunity to start exploring the frozen entrée section of you supermarket and also check out natural food stores, where you're sure to find brands such as Amy's, Moosewood, and Cedarlane (see page 303 for further suggestions). Their products are made with natural, often organic ingredients. For example, look for these three vegetarian offerings: Amy's Vegetable Lasagna, Cedarlane's Spinach and Monterey Jack Cheese Tamales, and Moosewood's Moroccan Stew. Start with these best bets and branch out from here.

Dinner: Indonesian chicken saté with peanut sauce and cucumber salad

The common peanut, which is really a legume and not a nut at all, provides a wide variety of vitamins and minerals. Eating peanuts is calories well spent! So enjoy some of this Indonesian chicken saté, traditionally served with a spicy peanut sauce. Be sure to also prepare the cucumber salad, just the right flavor note to have with the creamy peanut sauce.

Indonesian Chicken Saté: See page 244 for the recipe.

Brown rice: Cook according to the package instructions. Alternatively, look for precooked brown rice, packaged in portion-size sacks that only require reheating in boiling water.

Asian Cucumber Salad: See page 264 for the recipe.

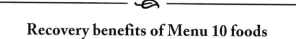

Recovery benefits of Menu 10 foods

▸ Beans are a reliable nondairy source of calcium as well as magnesium, which both lower the risk of osteoporosis, a possible outcome of long-term heavy drinking.

▸ Keeping high-quality and quick-to-fix frozen entrées on hand in your fridge is good insurance that you won't skip a meal and reach for a fast-food snack instead.

▸ Chicken is a source of vitamin B_6, sometimes deficient in persons who drink too much. This vitamin supports the nervous system, which chronic drinking can damage.

▸ Ginger offers many benefits as a digestive aid, an anti-inflammatory ally, and a subtle energizer.

▸ Brown rice is a source of folic acid, useful for replenishing this cancer-fighting B vitamin that drinking lots of coffee can deplete.

Menu 11

Breakfast: Yogurt-berry sundae

Having this sweet, creamy, and crunchy sundae for breakfast can lift the spirits, particularly if you have recently stopped drinking. Many recovering alcoholics soon develop a craving for sweets, a fix of sorts because consuming a carbohydrate such as sugar generates mellow feelings. A small serving of berries is a healthy way to satisfy your craving. See page 167 for the recipe.

Lunch: Gazpacho and Southwest chicken burger

Gazpacho soup requires no cooking; just chop, stir, and enjoy the super-fresh flavors. To complete the lunch, add a lean chicken burger. Shop for chicken patties with a Southwest flavor, great tasting with this gazpacho.

Mexican Gazpacho Soup: See page 214 for the recipe.

Southwest Chicken Burger: See page 259 for the recipe.

Dinner: Angel hair pasta with clam sauce and Italian-style garlic spinach

Angel Hair Pasta with Clam Sauce: Although the quickest way to make pasta with clam sauce is to use a canned sauce, nothing beats the clean flavor that fresh-cooked ingredients can give you. You'll want to keep sipping the sauce, it's so delicious, even while the pasta is still cooking! See page 184 for the recipe.

Italian-Style Spinach: And wait until you try this spinach. It is a pared-down version of a classic dish from Genoa that normally includes pine nuts and nutmeg. This shorter list of ingredients, which you're more likely to have on hand, delivers a mix of savory and sweet flavors. See page 206 for the recipe.

Recovery benefits of Menu 11 foods

▸ Raisins supply inulin, a special compound that helps the body rid itself of toxins produced in the gut, associated with drinking too much.

▸ Yogurt contains the friendly bacteria Lactobacillus acidophilus, which helps decrease those same gut toxins.

▸ Clams supply vitamin B_{12}, a nutrient that helps maintain the health of the nerves, specifically the nerve cell membranes. Drinking can interfere with the absorption of vitamin B_{12}.

▸ Spinach, like all green vegetables, contains chlorophyll, and at the center of each molecule of chlorophyll is magnesium. A magnesium deficiency, which is common in people who abuse alcohol, is thought to contribute to their higher risk of heart disease.

▸ Anchovies are an excellent source of omega-3 fish oils, essential foods for the brain.

Menu 12

Breakfast: Buckwheat pancakes with homemade fruit sauce

Add variety to your diet with these buckwheat pancakes, a fine option even if you're sensitive to wheat and need to avoid it. Buckwheat is actually the seed of a thistle! Instead of the usual maple syrup, top these pancakes with some homemade fruit syrup. The syrup can count as one of your servings of fruit for the day.

Pancake mixes: When shopping for a pancake mix, look for products made with whole wheat flour or buckwheat flour, to add nutrients and variety to your diet. Also stick to brands that have a relatively short ingredients list of ten or fewer natural-sounding items, with a minimum of sugar. Of course, you can always control all the ingredients by making pancakes from scratch, which isn't at all hard to do. Give it a try with the recipe on page 172.

Homemade Blueberry Syrup: See page 172 for the recipe.

Lunch: Meat loaf sandwich

Check the take-out counter of your supermarket and you'll likely find meat loaf as one of the standard offerings—a reliable dinner solution to keep in mind. But you can also turn meat loaf into a hefty sandwich. See page 258 for the recipe.

Other take-out counter items that can turn into sandwiches:

▸ Curried chicken salad on egg bread

▸ Marinated grilled salmon rolled into lettuce leaves

▸ Roasted turkey and coleslaw with Russian dressing on rye

Dinner: Grilled salmon on a bed of warm corn and lima bean salad

This combo, inspired by Southern cooking's succotash, assembles quickly. It includes fresh corn, lima beans—one of the most nutritious of the legumes, and summer savory, a less familiar herb that deserves a place in the kitchen for its delightfully earthy, green flavor. See page 222 for the recipe.

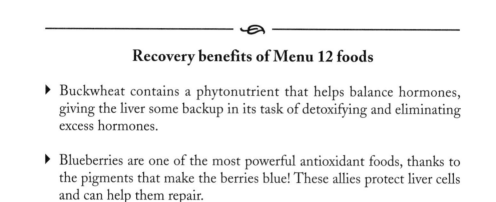

Recovery benefits of Menu 12 foods

▶ Buckwheat contains a phytonutrient that helps balance hormones, giving the liver some backup in its task of detoxifying and eliminating excess hormones.

▶ Blueberries are one of the most powerful antioxidant foods, thanks to the pigments that make the berries blue! These allies protect liver cells and can help them repair.

▶ Meat loaf makes a mouthwatering sandwich that can easily compete with the flavors of a fast-food burger, but with better-quality fixings. Check with your store manager for the best grade the market sells, whether frozen or ready-made, with a focus on lean meat and all-natural ingredients.

▶ Lima beans are food for the bones. These easy-to-digest legumes contain magnesium as well as copper, folic acid, and zinc, all needed for bone-building.

▶ Onions are an anti-inflammatory food; they help reduce chronic inflammation associated with many ailments that can result from heavy drinking, including gastritis, inflammation of the liver, and heart disease.

Menu 13

Breakfast: Diner breakfast: poached eggs, rye toast, and home fries

Enjoy the simple "good eats" of diner food in the comfort of your own home. Turn yourself into a short-order cook and make this breakfast your way, with healthy recovery ingredients.

Poached Eggs: Instead of having scrambled eggs, poach your eggs (see page 168 for the recipe). The aim is to minimize the exposure of the egg to high temperatures, which cause the cholesterol in the yolk to oxidize and become sticky. Frying an egg increases cholesterol's ability to produce artery-blocking plaque that can lead to a heart attack.

Rye toast: Try replacing wheat bread with woodsy-flavored rye toast. For maximum health (and taste), bring home pumpernickel bread, which is made with mostly rye flour, the chewier the better (a sign it contains whole grains). You also may want to try using a healthy butter substitute with a good mix of oils and no trans fats (such as Smart Balance) and, for a touch of sweetness, add a smear of all-fruit spread, in which the fruit itself, not white sugar, sweetens the product.

Home-Fries: See page 169 for the recipe.

Lunch: Curried "squash" soup with peanut butter and banana sandwich

While this may not be your standard combination, the flavors of squash, peanuts, and bananas go very well together. In fact, these same ingredients show up in African cooking, where they are combined in many time-honored dishes.

Peanut butter and banana sandwich: Peanuts are packed with vitamins and minerals and, when paired with a grain like wheat, form a complete protein, making this sandwich classic a great choice. Just make sure the brand of peanut butter you buy doesn't include added sugar and partially hydrogenated oils. Increase the health benefits of this sandwich by using whole wheat bread and letting the banana provide the sweetness, rather than using the usual jam. Make this sandwich with half a medium-size banana sliced into rounds.

Nearly Instant Curried "Squash" Soup: This soup is super simple to make because of some clever shortcuts, but tastes like you started from scratch. See page 213 for the recipe.

Alternatively, you might also opt for a boxed soup now increasingly available in supermarkets. These often have better flavor than canned. You'll likely find tomato and squash versions as well as corn chowder and ginger-carrot and potato. The advantage of these over canned soup is their easy access, just like pouring milk, and they close up tight to keep the unused portion fresh. Look on the ingredients list and you'll find many are made with soy milk, a good source of protein and nutrients and an option if you are lactose intolerant.

Dinner: Turkey sausage, polenta, and kale

Menu 4 gave you the chance to sample polenta for breakfast but Italians usually eat this traditional food for dinner. Polenta's mild flavor is the perfect backdrop for savory, rich turkey sausage and the assertive flavor of a dark, leafy green such as kale.

Turkey sausage: Select sausage that limits fat to around 15 percent per serving and contains a minimum of chemical additives. Avoid artificial colors and flavors. A good brand is Aidell's. You may pay a little more for a healthier version but it's worth the price. A dinner serving is about 4 ounces. Follow the package instructions and serve when heated through and browned.

Polenta: Follow the package instructions for this cornmeal mush, which is precooked and sold in a tube-shaped package. Just slice and fry in a skillet until lightly browned.

Sautéed Kale: See page 208 for the recipe.

Recovery benefits of Menu 13 foods

▸ Yukon Gold potatoes, thanks to their waxy texture, raise blood sugar less than do more starchy potatoes like russets and long whites used for baking. You can read more about how different foods affect blood sugar on pages 44–46.

▸ Pumpernickel bread is made with whole-grain, dark rye flour that retains most of the bran and germ, and is a source of magnesium and other trace minerals as well as the B vitamins folic acid, thiamine, and niacin.

▸ Pumpkin, as its orange color tells you, is a source of beta-carotene. This plant source of vitamin A is a nutrient that helps heal the tissues lining the digestive tract.

▸ Kale is a nondairy source of calcium as well as magnesium and cancer-fighting compounds. It deserves to be a regular on your table.

▸ Curry powder is a combination of any number of spices, each with its medicinal benefits. Commonly used spices include cardamom, which stimulates the release of bile; fennel, which is a digestive aid; and cloves, which promote digestion.

Menu 14

Breakfast: Dinner leftovers

There's nothing wrong nutritionally about eating dinner leftovers for breakfast if your meal the night before gave you a nice mix of carbs, protein, and fat. Such a mix of energy sources can keep your body and brain going until lunch. Or if dinner was spare but you have some healthy leftovers from a couple of lunches, such as soup or some rice pilaf and cooked vegetables, build a breakfast around these.

This breakfast suggestion assumes you cooked the turkey sausage and polenta of Menu 13 the day before. Reheat the sausage and polenta in the microwave oven or in a skillet with a bit of oil, and add a poached egg if you want this selection to taste more like breakfast and less like dinner revisited.

Lunch: Sautéed sweet red pepper salad and goat cheese

The tender crunch of these sautéed sweet red peppers goes beautifully with the creamy texture of goat cheese. Red peppers are also one of the best sources of antioxidants, beating out green peppers and containing more vitamin C than oranges. Once these peppers are cooked, they keep a couple of days in a sealed container, so you can assemble this lunch to take it to work. See page 208 for the recipe.

Dinner: Pork chops with sautéed onion and apple, plus sweet-and-sour red cabbage and egg noodles

The procedure for cooking these pork chops aims at keeping them moist, often an issue, especially when preparing the very thin chops sold in plastic-wrapped packages in markets. Thick chops are a better selection. Either thickness, these chops are great with sautéed onion and apple. Make a meal of this dish by heating up prepared sweet-and-sour cabbage and boiling egg noodles.

Pork Chops with Sautéed Onion and Apple: See page 256 for the recipe.

Sweet-and-sour red cabbage: Available bottled in the vegetable aisle of most grocery stores, this is very easy to prepare. Just open the bottle, put the cabbage in a pot, and warm over medium heat. Add a pinch or two of caraway seeds, if you wish.

Egg noodles: In a large pot of rapidly boiling water, add $1/2$ teaspoon of salt and 8 ounces of egg noodles to yield 4 servings. Cook, uncovered, stirring frequently, 8 to 10 minutes, or to desired tenderness. Drain and serve.

—————————————————— ✑ ——————————————————

Recovery benefits of Menu 14 foods

▸ Sweet red peppers offer the antioxidant beta-carotene and vitamin C, and also contain sulfur compounds that play a role in detox chemistry.

▸ Goat cheese may be better tolerated by people who cannot tolerate cheese made with cow's milk. Goat cheese is easier on digestion, as the fat globules in goat's milk tend to be smaller than those in cow's milk.

▸ Pork is a rich source of thiamine, one of the B vitamins that may become deficient due to drinking, as alcohol interferes with its absorption. Thiamine is a nutrient essential for brain function, necessary for communication between brain cells.

▸ Of their many benefits, apples are also a source of boron, a trace mineral that helps prevent osteoporosis.

▸ Cabbage contains compounds that keep detoxification processes moving ahead in the liver, taking part in both phases of the important two-step detox process.

Menu 15

Breakfast: Whole-grain breakfast cereal

Have whole-grain cereal for breakfast and you'll be adding to your intake of fiber, folic acid, magnesium, and vitamin E, while reducing your risk of digestion problems, diabetes, and heart disease. For a cold cereal, have Kashi's whole-grain puffs; for a hot cereal, make oatmeal. Alternatively, choose a bran cereal that is high in fiber, although it is not a true whole grain, as it's missing the germ and endosperm of the grain kernel. Suitable brands include Total and Grape-Nuts. Have these with milk and fruit for a satisfying and balanced breakfast. But use caution before you bring home whole-grain granola. Often, these mixes of dried fruit, nuts, seeds, and grains, while fortifying, are also full of calories and sugar. Check the ingredients list for the fat and sugar content and also for serving size before buying, and then make sure to keep portions moderate. A half cup of granola may be sufficient, whereas you can have at least a cup of whole-grain breakfast cereal.

Lunch: Salad bar minestrone soup

Minestrone means "big soup" in Italian and refers to a thick vegetable soup that likely contains both pasta and peas or beans. Although you can always buy canned minestrone, fresh minestrone delivers fuller flavor and your own choice of ingredients. This soup includes many of the special vegetables on the recovery shopping list and, by scooping them up from a salad bar, solves the problem of collecting a small amount of so many different kinds of ingredients. See page 215 for the recipe.

Dinner: Fish and fries with deli coleslaw

Junk food versions of fish and fries—those slivers of fish coated with spongy batter and potatoes cooked in stale oil you wouldn't want your pets to eat—are crossed off the recovery menu. But that's not to say you can never again enjoy succulent, meaty white fish coupled with the crunch of chips. Just prepare them yourself in a healthy way, using these two recipes. Start with the potatoes and, once the spuds are in the oven, begin to prepare the cod.

Oven-Baked "Fries": See page 210 for the recipe.

Crispy Cod Fillets: See page 233 for the recipe.

Recovery benefits of Menu 15 foods

▸ Vegetables and beans make up the bulk of minestrone soup, a good formula for an anticancer meal, according to studies of traditional diets from around the world that predominately serve plant foods.

▸ Soup is a good choice for a recovery meal, especially in the early days of abstinence, when you may have a weak stomach and have problems digesting food. Soup's well-cooked ingredients are easy to digest and the nutrients in the broth are readily absorbed.

▸ Cod is a low-fat source of protein. It's also a source of B vitamins.

▸ White potatoes with their skins give you potassium, which lowers blood pressure, and sweet potatoes are a top source of the antioxidant beta-carotene.

▸ Lemon juice and especially lemon peel contain the phytonutrient limonene, which helps remove toxins from the system—a good reason to squeeze some lemon juice on your fish and then nibble a little on the peel.

Menu 16

Breakfast: Meal in a muffin

The Everything Morning Muffin gives you protein, fat, and carbohydrates, plus fiber and plenty to chew on, including walnuts, raisins, oatmeal, and sunflower seeds. While a long list of ingredients are called for in the recipe (see page 166), these foods are all good staples to have in your kitchen.

Lunch: Beet soup and egg salad sandwich

Borscht, the beet soup that has sustained Russians and Poles for centuries, makes a fine lunch, served hot in winter and cold in summer. It's sold bottled in supermarkets. To add some protein to your lunch, while you're shopping, swing by the deli section and pick up a container of egg salad to make yourself an egg salad sandwich on whole-grain bread.

Beet soup: Heat the borscht in a saucepan or microwave oven and top with a generous spoonful of sour cream and a sprinkling of dill.

Dinner: Steak salad with sweet red peppers

This salad assembles fast when you start with bagged, prewashed and cut lettuce. These greens help fill you up on low-calorie ingredients and, of course, you can always add more vegetables to the salad, such as steamed asparagus and grilled mushrooms. See page 253 for the recipe.

Recovery benefits of Menu 16 foods

▸ Whole wheat contains over twenty vitamins and minerals, including B vitamins that maintain the adrenal glands, zinc for immunity, selenium to fight cancer, and magnesium and calcium for strong bones.

▸ Cinnamon, a mild sedative and painkiller, also has anticancer properties.

▸ Maple syrup raises blood sugar levels somewhat more slowly than refined white sugar does and it's also a source of potassium and calcium, unlike cane sugar that contains no nutrients at all.

▸ Sunflower seeds are packed with nutrients that can launch a sunflower plant—B vitamins, iron, potassium, selenium, and zinc, as well as relatively large amounts of protein.

▸ Beef is an excellent source of protein and easily absorbable iron. Having a small portion as in this salad lets you enjoy the flavor of steak while limiting saturated fat.

Menu 17

Breakfast: Breakfast in a muffin with Canadian bacon

Everything Breakfast Muffins, from Menu 16, stay fresh to eat the next day; if you crave a little variety, add Canadian bacon to this breakfast. This cut of bacon is more akin to ham than the sliced bacon you fry up in thin strips, and is leaner, but still delivers good pork flavor. It's precooked and, like ham, can be fried, baked, or enjoyed cold right from the package. Canadian bacon comes in slices and in cylindrical chunks. Figure on two thin slices, or 2 ounces, per serving.

Lunch: Chicken salad with avocado and papaya

You'll think you're suddenly at a fancy resort hotel when you serve yourself this colorful and elegant salad combo. Start with ready-made chicken salad from the deli section of the market. The avocado, calorie for calorie, provides high nutritional value as a source of potassium and B vitamins, needed to relieve stress, which can be one fallout of abstinence. And papaya aids digestion, which abusing alcohol may have weakened. See page 223 for the recipe.

Dinner: Turkish meatballs with traditional side dishes

Middle Eastern cooking offers its own unique palette of flavors, thanks to the spice-scented dishes of this region of the world, where trade routes crossed for centuries. These days as modern cultures intermingle, it's becoming easier and easier to find some Middle Eastern dishes ready-made, in specialty stores and even your local supermarket. Here's how to create a Turkish feast the easy way. Start with Turkish meatballs that go together as simply as meat loaf (see page 251 for the recipe).

Minted yogurt: Finely chop some of the remaining fresh mint used in the meatball recipe to yield 1 tablespoon of chopped mint. Mix with 1 cup of plain yogurt. Use as a sauce with the meatballs.

Hummus: This puree of chickpeas mixed with sesame paste (also known as tahini), lemon juice, and spices is widely available ready-made in the deli section of many markets. Hummus also makes a great dip for raw vegetables, a first-rate healthy snack.

Baba ghanoush: This savory eggplant appetizer is available ready-made in the deli section of many markets, as well as sold in jars and cans in Middle Eastern markets.

Cucumber and tomato salad: Peel one cucumber and remove the core and seeds from two tomatoes. Chop the vegetables into bite-size pieces. Dress with ⅓ cup of Basic Vinaigrette with Flaxseed Oil (see page 268 for the recipe).

Cinnamon Oranges: See page 275 for the recipe.

Recovery benefits of Menu 17 foods

▸ Canadian bacon, which is taken from the pork loin, delivers less fat than regular sliced bacon but still gives you the mouth-watering flavor of smoked meat.

▸ Avocados are a superior source of glutathione, an antioxidant manufactured in the body but also present in food. It's valued for the many important functions it performs, including maintaining a healthy liver.

▸ Papaya, when raw, contains papain, a living enzyme that aids digestion and decreases inflammation.

▸ Tahini, sesame seed paste, is a major ingredient in chickpea hummus. It is the peanut butter of Middle Eastern cooking, offering protein and many other nutrients, including the vitamins niacin and thiamine and the minerals calcium, potassium, magnesium, iron, and zinc.

▸ Orange zest contributes a special compound, cancer-fighting limonene, present in the oils within the orange peel.

Menu 18

Breakfast: Smoked salmon cream cheese on whole-grain bread

One of the delights of breakfast is looking forward to savoring smoked salmon cream cheese. The problem is this delicacy isn't always easy to find; it's invariably expensive and made with full-fat cream cheese. But there's nothing stopping you from making a lower-fat version at home. See page 173 for the recipe.

Lunch: Tabbouleh salad with Turkish dinner side dishes

This traditional Middle Eastern salad lets you enjoy a hearty dish without any cooking. The grain soaks in liquid for a few minutes and it's done. You then add the other ingredients, including lots of parsley and a touch of mint for a true Middle Eastern flair. Start with tabbouleh mix, following the package instructions, adding such ingredients as parsley, tomatoes, and olive oil. Or if you prefer to start from scratch for a salad with fresher taste, see page 176 for the recipe.

Leftover side dishes from Menu 17, such as hummus and baba ghanoush, are an excellent accompaniment to this hearty salad.

Dinner: Grilled halibut with tapenade, served with boiled potatoes and Greek-style green beans

This easily assembled dinner is inspired by Greek cooking. The traditional French condiment made with black olives, tapenade, makes a satisfying and quick sauce for any meaty fish. The two side dishes in the menu, the potatoes and the green beans, were chosen because these are also two key ingredients in Salade Niçoise. The recipes for these two vegetables call for more than the amount needed for dinner, giving you leftovers. Cook this dinner and you have an easy way to make a delicious salad the next day, the lunch in Menu 19.

Grilled Halibut with Tapenade: See page 237 for the recipe.

Boiled Potatoes: See page 210 for the recipe.

Greek-Style Green Beans: See page 209 for the recipe.

--------------------------- ∽ ---------------------------

Recovery benefits of Menu 18 foods

▶ Salmon or other fish at breakfast increases the likelihood you'll be eating your quota of two to three servings of fish per week, a prescription for health because of the fish oils, which are anti-inflammatory and help prevent blood clots.

▶ Parsley in the tabbouleh is a source of lutein, an antioxidant that goes to work in the eye, guarding against macular degeneration. Abusing alcohol can decrease the amount of lutein in the body.

▶ Tapenade, which is made with olives, gives you a rich source of proven heart-healthy monounsaturated fats.

▶ Green beans are a source of soluble fiber, which promotes the secretion of bile that carries toxins out of the system.

▶ Bulgur wheat is a whole grain and contains choline, a nutrient that promotes the flow of fat to and from the liver, helping to prevent the accumulation of fat in liver tissue and consequently fatty liver disease.

Menu 19

Breakfast: Oatmeal with poached gingered pears

Poached Pears Scented with Cardamom: Poached pears, an elegant dessert, are just as welcome at breakfast. Usually poached in wine, in this version the pears are cooked with ginger to enhance their flavor. These two foods also work together to ease digestion, which may need some help especially in the early stages of recovery. See page 276 for the recipe.

Oatmeal: Follow the package instructions for cooking the desired number of servings. Put the oatmeal into individual bowls. Top with 1 teaspoon of butter or butter substitute per serving and add three or four gingered pear slices to each. Add $^1/_2$ cup of 2% milk per serving, if desired.

Lunch: Salade Niçoise with pesto baguette

The classic version of this tuna salad, called Salade Niçoise, includes tiny olives de Nice, sweet peppers, and hard-boiled eggs. This version is less complicated and less pricey.

Enjoy it with another south-of-France specialty, pesto, a healthy mix of basil, pine nuts, cheese, garlic, and olive oil, which you can spread on French bread like butter. Make sure to buy chunk light tuna, which has lower levels of mercury than albacore tuna. A shortcut for making this salad is to use some of the extra potatoes and green beans cooked for Menu 18's dinner. You'll find recipes for these on pages 210 and 209, respectively.

Tuna Salade Niçoise: See page 223 for the recipe.

Pesto baguette: Start with a baguette loaf of French bread. Cut slices, crosswise, almost to the bottom of the loaf and spread each slice with prepared pesto. Use about 2 tablespoons pesto, per 12-inch length of baguette. Wrap in foil and heat for 10 minutes in an oven preheated to 350°F. If you only have access to a microwave oven, if you've brought this lunch to your office, heat a portion of the pesto bread on low for 10 seconds to warm and still maintain the bread's texture.

Dinner: Frozen chicken enchilada with pinto beans and Mexican rice

You don't need to go out to your favorite Mexican restaurant to enjoy an enchilada dinner complete with beans and rice. You can easily make this recovery-friendly version at home. Start with a healthy brand of frozen enchiladas, following package instructions for preparation. The addition of the sides below will create a tasty, filling meal.

Red pinto beans: Instead of canned refried beans, which are cooked in hot oil, use canned whole red pinto beans and stew them with some oregano and garlic for extra flavor.

Mexican Rice: All you need is a tomato, a clove of garlic, and a bit of onion to turn plain rice into a colorful and tasty dish with flavors from south of the border. See page 181 for the recipe.

Recovery benefits of Menu 19 foods

▶ Pears raise blood sugar more slowly than many other fruits do, helping control blood sugar levels, an issue often associated with abusing alcohol.

▶ Tuna is a source of the fish oils DHA and EPA that protect against heart disease and nourish brain tissue, and are essential for recovery.

▶ Ginger is a warming spice that both stimulates the circulation and eases digestion.

▶ Frozen chicken enchiladas waiting for you in your fridge are a fast-food option that works for recovery because, by selecting a healthy brand, you give yourself an easy-to-prepare, nourishing meal.

▶ Pinto beans are high in folate, a B vitamin that is poorly absorbed when drinking has disrupted the normal workings of the digestive tract.

Menu 20

Breakfast: Waffle Danish

Frozen Waffle Fantasy: If you're in the mood for a cheese Danish, but aren't looking forward to eating the white flour and white sugar in the usual item, don't despair. You can still enjoy a sensuous culinary treat for breakfast, the contrast of something warm and crunchy with a topping that is sweet, cool, and rich, with this healthy waffle combo. See page 168 for the recipe.

Lunch: Herb frittata

A frittata is an egg dish that starts out with the same ingredients as an omelet, but the ingredients are mixed with the eggs rather than folded inside. The procedure for cooking a frittata is a little more involved, but a slice of leftover frittata also makes a great no-cook meal the next day. You first cook the eggs in a skillet and then finish the dish by baking the eggs in the oven. If you want to take some frittata to the office, make this dish the day before. Frittata keeps well in the refrigerator overnight and tastes excellent the next day. See page 171 for the Herb Frittata recipe.

To vary the frittata for the next day's breakfast, serve with Persian-style yogurt which is thickened and scented with mint. You'll find the recipe for Yogurt Cheese on page 265.

Dinner: Seafood supper

Mediterranean Fish Stew: This all-in-one-pot fish stew is a time saver and full of flavor. I guarantee you'll be making this dish again and again. See page 235 for the recipe.

Recovery benefits of Menu 20 foods

▸ All-fruit preserves are a delicious and healthier alternative to jellies and jams made with sugar, because the sweetener in all-fruit preserves is natural fruit sugar, which raises blood sugar more slowly.

▸ Eggs supply selenium, a trace mineral that works with vitamin E to enhance its antioxidant action.

▸ Dairy products like ricotta cheese offer a source of protein as well as calcium, one of the minerals that is sometimes deficient in those who abuse alcohol.

▸ Carrots, one of the foods that can raise blood sugar quickly, is just fine to include in a recovery diet when eaten in moderate quantities. Enjoy them as a side dish and added to this day's herb frittata.

▸ Tomatoes, when they're cooked and consumed with some fat, are extra good for you because eating them this way increases the absorption of their anticancer component lycopene.

Menu 21

Breakfast: Herb frittata with yogurt cheese

This make-ahead breakfast combines yesterday's lunch frittata with a topping of yogurt cheese, also known as Greek yogurt and, in the Middle East, *lebnah*. After it has been drained for a few hours, the thickened yogurt can be enjoy as is, mixed with sweet and savory flavorings, or added to cooked dishes. For this breakfast, it's mixed with mint and a touch of olive oil, but you can also reserve some and serve it with today's curry dinner.

Yogurt Cheese: Because this yogurt requires straining overnight, plan on starting to prepare this yogurt cheese the day before you'll want it. See page 265 for the recipe.

Lunch: Crab cakes

Look for crab cakes frozen in the freezer section of markets and freshly made in fish stores. Shellfish is very low in saturated fat yet a source of healing fish oils. And crab is low in cholesterol and supplies selenium, a trace mineral required by the liver to detoxify unwanted compounds. Enjoy these luxurious fish cakes when you're relaxing on a day off from work.

To prepare: Heat the crab cakes according to the package instructions, making sure a slightly crunchy, golden crust develops. Then dress up the crab cakes with any of the following:

▸ Deli coleslaw, wedge of lemon

▸ Bed of mixed baby lettuce leaves, avocado slices, Russian dressing

▸ Asian cucumber salad from Menu 10 (page 264), pickled ginger slices

▸ Dollop of low-fat sour cream topped with a dusting of black caviar

Dinner: Curry in a hurry

As life becomes more global, even once-exotic products like curry sauces now sit comfortably on supermarket shelves next to Chinese water chestnuts and bottles of Mexican chile peppers. Most curry sauces are only moderately spicy if that, but you can always add to the heat with additional curry powder. You can also expand this dish into a feast with many Indian side dishes based on lentils, spinach, eggplant, or chickpeas, now sold packaged in handy aluminum foil packets. All you need do is pop these into boiling water to heat, remove from the pot, tear open the bag, and serve. Read labels and make sure to select a product that's not loaded with salt and saturated fats. Look in natural food stores for such brands as Tandoor Chef and Amy's for tasty Indian side-dishes. And don't forget the mango chutney and the raita, a classic Indian condiment that combines yogurt and spices.

Chicken Curry: See page 245 for the recipe.

Spiced yogurt: Start with a cup of yogurt or some of the remaining yogurt cheese from this menu's breakfast. Peel and remove the seeds from a 2-inch length of cucumber and grate the cucumber to yield ¼ cup. Season with ¼ teaspoon of cumin. As a variation, use a teaspoon of minced fresh mint leaves along with the cumin.

Recovery benefits of Menu 21 foods

▶ Yogurt with live cultures of bacteria encourages the synthesis of the B vitamins biotin, folic acid, and B_{12}, and also increases the absorption of calcium and magnesium.

▶ Crab meat is an excellent source of zinc, often needed in recovery because the way the body metabolizes alcohol uses up supplies. Drinking also decreases zinc's absorption and increases its excretion.

▶ Peas deliver fiber, which helps maintain normal function of the intestinal wall, helping prevent leaky gut syndrome.

▶ Pecans are high in unsaturated fats and provide some fiber and a good dose of vitamin E.

▶ Turmeric, one of the spices in Indian curry, contains a compound called *curcumin* that inhibits the activation of carcinogens while increasing detoxification of others.

Having a Little Something in between Meals

There's room in recovery eating for a snack between meals. Giving yourself a little something can even be therapeutic if you're having problems with blood sugar, since eating a snack that gives you some protein and fat can help stabilize blood glucose. When blood sugar begins to dip a few hours after a meal, which can suddenly lower your energy and mood, take that as a signal that it's time to have a bite. Between-meal noshing is also a great way to give yourself certain nutritious foods that may not show up enough in your normal meals, such as nuts and seeds as well as fruits and vegetables. Reaching for a snack may also make it less likely you'll reach for junk food, or worse, a drink, if the underlying need is to use up nervous energy and quiet nerves. Nibbling throughout the day, using food rather than a drink, may also satisfy an oral need to put something in your mouth, a habit that some former drinkers may still have. Keep healthy snack foods handy, at home, in the car, and at the office, so they are ready when you need them.

Of course, snacking doesn't mean reverting to those probably none-too-healthy tidbits you used to munch on in your drinking days—the typical bar assortment of deep-fried, super-salty snacks. Stock up on healthy snack foods as you would plan for any other meal and create your own snacks with recovery ingredients. You can feel pleased that you're doing something good for your health while enjoying a little bite. Here are some suggestions.

▸ Spiced and Toasted Nuts (see page 266 for the recipe)

▸ Garlic-Onion Dip (see page 263 for the recipe)

▸ Store-bought hummus and whole-grain crackers

▸ Raw recovery vegetables such as slices of sweet peppers, broccoli and cauliflower florets, cherry tomatoes, carrot and cucumber sticks, plus dip (Garlic-Onion Dip or hummus)

▸ Celery stuffed with goat cheese

▸ Peanut butter spread on apple wedges

▸ Recovery fruit such as slices of cantaloupe, sliced papaya and mango, orange segments, sliced peaches, pears and apples, berries such as blueberries and strawberries, and such dried fruits as raisins, prunes, and dates

▸ Frozen grapes

▸ Trail mix, ready-made or homemade, such as a mixture of walnuts, dried cranberries, and toasted whole-grain cereal such as Kashi brand; almonds, sunflower seeds, and raisins

▸ Plain yogurt and fresh fruit

▸ Whole-grain pretzels with mustard

▸ Popcorn

▸ Ice pops made with unsweetened fruit juice

▸ Whole-grain crackers and cheddar cheese

▸ Creamed herring on crackers

▸ Roasted nuts

Care for Some Dessert?

You've probably noticed that the menus in this chapter don't include dessert. Since desserts, at least really yummy ones, contain lots of fat and sugar, they don't strictly belong in the recovery diet. But of course there will be times when you'll want something rich and sweet at the end of a meal. Like many people who have had a problem with alcohol, in the early phase of abstinence, you may begin to crave sweets even though you probably did not have a sweet tooth in your drinking days. You may need the feel-good fix that carbs produce. Carbohydrates increase the production of serotonin, a brain chemical that gives a person a sense of well-being. Of course, your desire for something sweet isn't a license to binge on sugar whenever you wish. You may have a day when you can't stop yourself, but the goal is to rely on wholesome carbs like whole grains, an alternative way to generate that serotonin. Having sufficient protein in your diet and controlling swings of blood sugar can also help. (You can read more about controlling blood sugar on pages 44–46.)

Of course if you aren't someone who can stop with one cookie, then try not to start! For something sweet, experiment with having fruit instead, a good way to make sure you eat your daily quota. Enjoy one of the fruits recommended for recovery (see page 98) in season with all its full, ripe flavor. Buy some organic strawberries and dip them in low-fat sour cream. Poach pears with a touch of cinnamon and nutmeg, following the instructions on page 276, in the poaching liquid. Bake an apple, following the recipe on page 275. Top an apple with a spoonful of vanilla ice cream for a shortcut to the taste of apple pie à la mode. And for more sweet things, consult the desserts section in chapter 6.

What to Drink Now That You're Not Drinking?

This isn't the wasteland of options that you might imagine now that beer, wine, and stronger substances are no longer a choice and you're even cutting back on caffeine. As you'll discover in the beverage section of chapter 6, you can mix up all sorts of fruit juice and herbal tea combinations with ingredients such as yogurt and mint to give you a taste of sweet and quench your thirst. There are even great flavored coffee substitutes that offer a caffeine-free way of enjoying the wonderfully bitter taste of java.

Quench your thirst whenever you need to. You'll probably be thirsty during your first weeks of recovery. Drinking leaves the body dehydrated, since alcohol is a diuretic. Liquids, especially water, are also a good flush for any alcohol and the toxic by-products of alcohol metabolism that remain in the system even after abstinence begins.

But be warned. Don't mess with your mind or your senses and concoct beverages reminiscent of alcoholic drinks. If you loved Blood Marys, maybe you shouldn't be sipping V-8 juice, lest you be tempted to add a shot of vodka. You may also need to avoid using wineglasses and familiar cocktail glasses, even though filled with tamer liquids, in case these visual cues trigger a desire for something stronger. And don't kid yourself about having a nonalcoholic beer or wine. These beverages can contain trace amounts of alcohol and even the sight of the typical shape of the bottle or a whiff of these beverages may trigger brain chemistry that can reactivate cravings.

Eating Well When Eating Out

The basic guidelines for healthy eating at home still apply when eating out: stay away from highly processed and refined foods like white flour and white sugar as much as possible, skip the deep-fried numbers, and stay away from junk food. Fortunately these days, most places from fancy dining joints to fast-food outlets are making an attempt at offering healthy eating options. The following ordering suggestions will turn you into a savvy customer.

▸ Skip the bread basket and order soup and/or salad instead. To avoid saturated fats, your best soup options are vegetable, bean, and lentil, and broth-based rather than creamed soups. As for salad, if you know the restaurant drowns its salads in dressing, ask for it on the side and add with discretion. You can also ask for vinegar and oil to dress your salad simply.

▸ Order protein lower in saturated fat—chicken, turkey, and seafood rather than beef, pork, and lamb. And avoid these foods when prepared with cream-based sauces in such dishes as chicken or turkey à la King, shrimp Newburg, and creamy clam chowder.

▶ Replace potatoes and rice with a vegetable, but stay away from items such as creamed spinach and deep-fried onion rings, to limit fat.

▶ If you want a recovery meal and you're vegetarian, in a regular restaurant, try ordering a vegetable platter even if it's not on the menu. Cooks in some restaurants will be willing and able to assemble a variety of that day's vegetable side dishes to produce a very tasty meal.

▶ Stay away from all fried foods.

▶ Remember that the salads at fast-food eateries may appear to be healthy alternatives to the burger and fries but the dressing can deliver as many calories.

▶ Opt for water or iced tea with your meal, rather than sugary fruit juice or colas. And don't let the waiter automatically pour you a cup of coffee when you first sit down and then keep refilling it throughout the meal.

▶ If the dish you've ordered comes with a buttery sauce, ask for it to be served on the side so you can control how much you're eating but still have some to enjoy the flavor.

▶ If you want something sweet, choose fruit for dessert, or order one dessert and split it four ways.

▶ Of course, avoid all dishes made with wine, those that have *au vin* in their name, and anything that comes flambéed, and feel free to ask the waiter point blank which dishes are cooked with some form of alcohol.

Go Native

Restaurants that specialize in the native cooking of a particular country or region are often a good bet because the traditional dishes they serve typically contain an array of healthy ingredients. Such foods have withstood the test of time, able to sustain the health of populations over hundreds if not thousands of years. Now, I'm not talking about sugar-coated, deep-fried Sweet-and-Sour Chicken and Navajo fried bread. The traditional ingredients I'm referring to are all the beans and lentils, spices and herbs, grilled and baked chicken, fish and meats, vegetables, nuts, and so forth that are mainstays of these cuisines.

Here are some dishes to order in restaurants that serve traditional foods:

Mexican restaurants. While the cheese, full-fat sour cream, tortilla chips, and refried beans aren't the healthiest, there are plenty of recovery-friendly dishes available. Try fish tacos, guacamole, salsa, stewed beans rather than refried beans, chicken fajita, grilled and baked fish, corn tortillas, which are whole grain and higher in calcium than flour tortillas, which are made with white flour, and cactus salad (nopales).

Italian. If you refrain from selecting cream-based sauces and lots of Parmesan, you'll find many Italian dishes that are delicious and good for you. Some examples are: vegetable and bean antipasto dishes, prosciutto and melon, minestrone soup, green salad with oil and vinegar dressing, chicken scaloppine, pasta with tomato sauce or clam sauce, sautéed spinach, and broccoli rabe.

Chinese. You can avoid deep-fried selections and choose dishes that are pan or stir fried or steamed. Try shrimp or chicken with mixed vegetables, egg drop soup without the fried noodles, Buddha's Delight featuring mixed sautéed vegetables and tofu, or steamed whole fish. Ask for brown rice instead of white.

Japanese. While the deep-fried tempura may be tempting, many other Japanese dishes are extremely healthy for you, such as sushi, meat and chicken teriyaki, grilled fish, whole soybeans (edamame), miso soup, vinegared vegetable condiments such as cucumber and pickled ginger, and soba noodles.

Middle Eastern. While you'll want to go easy with the piles of white rice pilaf often served with these meals, there are plenty of Middle Eastern options to enjoy guilt free. Try hummus, baba ghanoush, yogurt dip, meat and chicken kebabs, and tomato and cucumber salad.

Indian. Although some Indian dishes are cream-based, the following options are good choices for recovery eating: chicken tandoori; the cucumber and yogurt condiment called *raita*; chicken curry in yogurt sauce; *dal*, which is made with lentils; and chickpeas, pureed spinach, cauliflower, okra; and, for a sweet finish, mango *lassi*.

As you can tell by reading this chapter, recovery eating is flexible enough that you can adapt it to your particular way of life, whether you mostly eat at home, have lunch weekdays at work, travel a lot, or simply choose to eat out. You also don't have to be limited to the twenty-one menus. They're meant to be a starting point for eating better as you find your way into sober living. But as you become comfortable with the menus, feel free to adapt and move beyond these. Explore and invent your own. All sorts of dishes can work for recovery, and that's what you'll find in the next chapter.

6 EATING MORE HOME-COOKED MEALS
Recipes for Recovery

THIS CHAPTER IS A mini-cookbook of recipes for recovery. Many of the recipes are for the dishes recommended in chapter 5, quick and easy things to cook that are featured in the twenty-one recovery menus, whereas other recipes take you into new territory. This chapter is divided into recipe sections, each featuring a particular type of food or meal, such as Soups or Breakfast Dishes.

All the recipes feature important recovery foods, discussed in chapter 4 —ingredients that can do their part in repairing damage to various body systems caused by drinking too much alcohol. For example, Egg Drop Soup and Carrot Slaw help the liver mend, Down-South Okra and Baked Apples with Cranberry Chutney improve digestion, Chicken Curry and Fresh Salsa are good for the heart, and Grilled Salmon on Toasted Corn and Lima Bean Salad helps the brain recover. Don't worry, you don't have to be a wizard chef to prepare such dishes. For the most part, the recovery recipes rely on simple skills: boiling in water, sautéing foods in a pan with a little oil, or putting something in the oven to bake. And for some recipes, you need only know how to handle a paring knife and use a can opener!

This chapter will inspire you to expand beyond the foods you may currently eat. Recipes that call for certain specialty ingredients, such as Medjool dates and kalamata olives, may send you to gourmet and ethnic food shops, where you'll discover other healthy goodies as you browse. And buying organic may take you into the new and fascinating world of natural foods stores. Many ingredients you have never used before may be found right at your local grocer's, such as in the fresh produce aisles. You have much to look forward to as you explore this chapter.

Cook with Organic Ingredients as Much as You Can

Goal 7 of the nutrition program, eating more organic foods, will probably have you shopping at a health food store or one of the natural food emporiums, such as Whole Foods, if your usual grocery store or farmers' market doesn't offer them. Other places to check out: mega-supermarkets and gourmet grocers are carrying more and more organic goods, such superstores as Wal-Mart are beginning to heed customers' requests to stock organic groceries, and online sellers will be glad to ship nonperishibles to your door (see Healthy Food Resources, pages 300–307).

The recipes in this chapter don't call specifically for organic ingredients, but use them whenever possible. Especially go out of your way to cook with the following:

▶ Organic butter and other dairy products
▶ Organic citrus when a recipe calls for orange zest or lemon peel
▶ Organic fruits and vegetables listed in chapter 4, page 98.

Breakfast Dishes

The Recipes:

Basic Breakfast Shake ⓦ
Everything Morning Muffin ⓦ
Yogurt-Berry Sundae
Frozen Waffle Fantasy
Poached Eggs ⓦ
Home Fries
Mexican Poached Eggs
Spinach-Egg Scramble
Herb Frittata
Whole Wheat Pancakes ⓦ
Homemade Blueberry Syrup ⓦ
Smoked Salmon Cream Cheese

Having a good breakfast, a cornerstone of recovery eating, is something to really look forward to when you start with these tasty breakfast dishes. They give you protein and lots of nutrients to repair the body and also provide fuel for the day. Some, such as the breakfast shake, can be prepared quickly before heading out the door; others, for example the muffins, are made ahead; and then there are such dishes as Mexican Poached Eggs, for when you have a bit of time to cook and savor what you've made.

Basic Breakfast Shake 🐾
(Menu 7)

If you have a blender, a nourishing breakfast is only two or three minutes away with this shake and its many variations (see page 124 for details on these), a far better option than oversweetened cereals and sugary breakfast-food products that give you quick energy and then let you drop.

YIELD: 2 SERVINGS

2 cups fruit, such as mango, peeled, pitted, and diced
1 cup low-fat yogurt
1 cup 2% milk, filtered water, or ice cubes

Flavorings and healthy add-ins such as fresh mint and protein powder (See page 124 for more suggestions.) (optional)

1. Put the fruit, yogurt, and milk (or water or ice cubes) in a blender and mix until thoroughly combined, about 15 seconds.

2. Add chosen flavorings and any other ingredients and blend again, about 5 seconds.

3. Pour into two glasses and sip your breakfast.

Everything Morning Muffin 🐾
(Menu 16)

When you don't have time to cook breakfast, grab one of these muffins. They're chock full of whole grains, eggs, milk, nuts, seeds, and fruit for a satisfying mini-meal.

YIELD: 12 MUFFINS

Dry ingredients:
2 cups rolled oats
1 cup whole wheat pastry flour
1/2 cup chopped walnuts
1/2 cup raisins
1/2 cup sunflower seeds
2 tablespoons baking powder
1 teaspoon ground cinnamon or allspice
1/2 teaspoon salt

Wet ingredients:
2 eggs
1/2 cup milk
1/2 cup applesauce
1/2 cup pure maple syrup
1/4 cup unrefined safflower oil

Special equipment: muffin tin for twelve muffins, twelve 2 1/2-inch paper baking cups

Preheat the oven to 375°F.

1. Put all the dry ingredients in a large bowl and mix to combine.

2. Put the eggs in a second bowl and scramble with a fork. Add the milk, applesauce, maple syrup, and oil, and mix.

3. Pour the wet ingredients into the dry ingredients and stir just enough to thoroughly moisten the dry ingredients.

4. Line a muffin pan with the paper baking cups and spoon batter into the twelve cups. Bake the muffins in the preheated oven for 25 to 30 minutes, until golden on top.

5. Transfer the muffins to a cooling rack or turn the muffins upside down in the pan to cool the bottoms and keep the tops moist. Enjoy warm and on the next day. Any remaining muffins can be frozen; defrost and reheat in a toaster oven, not a microwave, to retain the muffins' texture.

Yogurt–Berry Sundae
(Menu 11)

This sundae benefits digestion, thanks to the yogurt, and the berries fight cancer.

YIELD: 2 SERVINGS

1 banana
1 cup berries, fresh or frozen, plus some reserved for garnish

1 cup low-fat yogurt
$1/2$ cup Grape-Nuts cereal or granola

1. Slice the banana. If using frozen berries, microwave for 15 seconds to partially defrost. Cover the bottoms of two sundae dishes or stemmed glasses with half of the bananas and berries.

2. Top with half of the yogurt.

3. Sprinkle with some of the Grape-Nuts.

4. Add the remaining fruit and then the remaining yogurt.

5. Top with the remaining cereal and garnish with the reserved fruit.

Frozen Waffle Fantasy
(Menu 20)

This recipe would normally call for vanilla extract, which can be off limits to someone in recovery since a large percentage of this extract consists of alcohol. But there is an alternative, alcohol-free version on the market: Cook's brand pure vanilla powder is vanilla bean in a dextrose base. When vanilla extract is called for in a recipe, simply substitute an equal amount of the powder. See page 307 for the Cook's Web address.

YIELD: 4 SERVINGS
3 tablespoons low-fat ricotta cheese
$^1/_4$ teaspoon vanilla powder
1 frozen whole wheat waffle, or
    gluten-free, brown rice waffle
1 tablespoon all-fruit preserves

1. Put the ricotta in a small bowl and mix with the vanilla powder.

2. Toast the waffle and, when it's ready, smear a tablespoon of preserves on the waffle and then add the ricotta on top. Enjoy!

Poached Eggs 🥚
(Menu 13)

The healthiest way to eat eggs is poached, cooked with no fat and exposed to only low heat.

YIELD: 2 SERVINGS
1 teaspoon white vinegar
1 teaspoon salt
2 eggs

1. Put about an inch of water in a deep skillet and bring to a boil. Add the vinegar and salt, and lower the heat until the water barely bubbles.

2. Break the egg into a bowl and gently slide into the water. Cover and cook for 3 to 5 minutes, until the yolk has filmed over and the white has set. Use a slotted spoon to remove the eggs.

Home Fries
(Menu 13)

A cut above your standard diner fries, these delicious potatoes are not a tangle of some shredded processed product, but hand-sliced potatoes sautéed with onions and sweet peppers. Start with cooked potatoes, to save time in the morning and as a way to use up leftovers.

YIELD: 4 SERVINGS

1 pound cooked round red or Yukon Gold potatoes
1 small onion
1/2 green bell pepper, seeded
2 tablespoons unrefined safflower oil
Pinch of paprika

1. Slice the potatoes. Trim and chop the onion and bell pepper into bite-size pieces.

2. Heat the oil in a large skillet over medium heat. Add the potatoes, onion, pepper, and paprika.

3. Cook, turning occasionally with a spatula, until the onion softens and the potatoes turn golden, 12 to 15 minutes. Season with salt and pepper, and serve.

Mexican Poached Eggs
(Menu 5)

This easy go-together is a quick version of huevos rancheros. It gives you a delicious way to start the day with a serving of vegetables, thanks to the tomatoes, plus whole grains in the corn tortillas.

YIELD: 4 SERVINGS

1 (28-ounce) can stewed tomatoes
8 eggs
8 corn tortillas
Prepared salsa

1. Whirl the stewed tomatoes in a blender or food processor to give them the texture of a sauce, leaving some small chunks.

2. Put the tomato sauce into a skillet and cook, uncovered, for 10 minutes until the sauce is reduced somewhat.

(recipe continues, next page)

3. Crack the eggs, one at a time, onto a saucer and carefully slide them into the hot tomato sauce, taking care that the yolk does not break. Cover the skillet with a lid or foil and allow the eggs to poach very gently until set, 6 to 8 minutes.

4. While the eggs are cooking, warm the tortillas.

5. Spoon the eggs and sauce into individual bowls, two eggs per serving. Serve immediately with the warmed tortillas and salsa.

Note: An easy way to "steam" tortillas is to heat them in a microwave oven. Stack three on a plate, sprinkling a few drops of water on each before laying down the next, and heat for 30 seconds.

Spinach-Egg Scramble
(Menu 9)

A scramble made with the same ingredients as for an omelet gives you the same flavors but without the fussing. Better to make sure you eat than worry about some tricky technique.

YIELD: 1 SERVING

1 handful spinach leaves from a bag of washed and chopped spinach	Salt and pepper
2 eggs	1 teaspoon butter substitute, such as Smart Balance Buttery Spread, or
1 tablespoon milk	olive oil

1. Put a cup of water in a small saucepan and bring to a boil.

2. Add the spinach and a pinch of salt and cook, covered, for about 1 minute, until the leaves are tender and bright green. Drain through a sieve and use a spoon to press all the remaining liquid from the spinach. Transfer to a work surface and chop the spinach.

3. Beat the eggs in a bowl. Add the spinach and milk, and season with salt and pepper. Stir to combine.

4. Heat the butter in an omelet pan over medium heat, swirling it around the pan. Add the egg mixture and lower the heat to low. Cook for 1 minute, stirring frequently, just until the eggs have lost their runny quality. Serve immediately.

Herb Frittata
(Menu 20)

Parsley is considered a cleansing herb and scallions, like other onions, dampen inflammation.

YIELD: 4 SERVINGS
4 sprigs fresh parsley
4 sprigs fresh dill
2 scallions
6 eggs
Salt and pepper
2 tablespoons extra-virgin olive oil

Preheat the oven to 350°F.

1. Remove the stems of the parsley and dill, and finely chop the leaves of both herbs. Trim the scallions and cut crosswise into ¼-inch pieces.

2. Break the eggs into a medium-size bowl and beat with a fork. Stir the parsley, dill, and scallions into the eggs. Season with salt and pepper.

3. Coat the sides and bottom of a large, ovenproof skillet, preferably nonstick, with the oil and place over medium heat. When the oil is hot, pour the egg mixture into the skillet. Lower the heat to medium-low. Cook undisturbed until the bottom of the frittata is firm, about 7 minutes.

4. Put the skillet in the preheated oven. Bake for 10 minutes and test for doneness, being careful not to overcook. The top of the frittata should still be a bit runny, as the eggs will continue to set once removed from the heat. If necessary, bake for another 5 minutes.

5. Making sure to wear heatproof oven mitts, take the skillet out of the oven and place on a heatproof work surface. Loosen the frittata with a spatula and, again wearing mitts, use the handle of the skillet to tip the pan so that the frittata slides gently onto a serving platter. Frittatas are also great for breakfast. Serve with some cinnamon-flavored fresh orange slices (see page 275).

Note: Also try these other frittata filling options: diced cooked potatoes, diced cooked carrots, small chunks cooked zucchini, defrosted frozen peas, and watercress.

Whole Wheat Pancakes 𝒲
(Menu 12)

Made with pastry flour, these pancakes are light and fluffy and the whole grain gives you maximum nutrients.

YIELD: 4 SERVINGS

2 cups whole wheat pastry flour
1 tablespoon baking powder
1 teaspoon ground cinnamon
$1/2$ teaspoon salt

1 egg
$1^1/_2$–2 cups 2% milk
3–4 tablespoons unrefined safflower
    oil, plus oil for greasing the griddle

Preheat the oven to 200°F.

1. Preheat a griddle or large skillet over medium-low heat while you prepare the batter.

2. Mix together in a large bowl the flour, baking powder, cinnamon, and salt.

3. In another large bowl, combine the egg, milk, and 2 tablespoons of the oil. Pour the liquid ingredients into the dry and mix until just moistened. The batter should pour easily from a ladle or measuring cup. To thin the batter, add more milk.

4. Grease the hot griddle with 1 to 2 teaspoons of the oil. When the oil shimmers, ladle the batter onto the griddle to form pancakes of your desired size. Cook for 2 to 4 minutes, until the pancakes are cooked on the bottom. Flip and cook until the second side is lightly browned. Add additional oil for each batch of pancakes.

5. Transfer the pancakes to a platter and keep in a warm oven, 200°F, while other pancakes cook. Serve with the warm Homemade Blueberry Syrup.

Homemade Blueberry Syrup 𝒲
(Menu 12)

This fruit syrup beats out pancake syrup by a mile, when it comes to health benefits. Blueberries contain a whole collection of antioxidants that work together to protect body tissues, in particular protecting the brain from damage.

YIELD: 2 CUPS

1 tablespoon cornstarch
$3/4$ cup blueberry juice or apple juice
12 ounces fresh or frozen blueberries,
   thawed
2 tablespoons pure maple syrup
Pinch of ground cinnamon

1. In a small bowl, combine the cornstarch with 1 tablespoon of cold water, stirring with a fork. Set aside.

2. Put the fruit juice, blueberries, maple syrup, and cinnamon in a small saucepan and warm over medium heat until the sauce simmers.

3. Add the cornstarch mixture and continue to cook, stirring frequently, for about 3 minutes, until the sauce thickens. Prepare the syrup in the morning if you have a few minutes or prepare the day before and reheat at breakfast time.

Smoked Salmon Cream Cheese
(Menu 18)

This deli classic is usually eaten on toasted bagels, but it also tastes just right on chewy whole-grain pumpernickel, which has much less of an effect on blood sugar and is healthier for recovery.

YIELD: SIX 2-OUNCE SERVINGS

1 (4-ounce) package smoked salmon
1 (8-ounce) package low-fat cream
   cheese

1. To make the salmon and cream cheese easier to process, cut the salmon into a few big pieces and break the cheese into large chunks.

2. Put the salmon and cheese in a food processor fitted with a metal blade. Pulse the processor about six times, just enough to combine the two ingredients. When properly mixed, there should be small bits of salmon still visible in the cream cheese and the cheese should have a fluffy texture. Overprocessing will create a gummy texture.

Whole Grains and Pasta

The Recipes:

Tabbouleh
Green Bell Peppers Stuffed with Brown Rice and Spices
Quinoa Pilaf
Wild Rice Pilaf with Pecans 🅦
Breakfast Polenta 🅦
Barley Scented with Summer Savory 🅦
Mexican Rice
Kasha with Mushrooms and Walnuts
Pasta Primavera with Pesto 🅦
Angel Hair Pasta with Clam Sauce
Pasta with Fresh Peas and Prosciutto
Buckwheat Soba Noodles in Chinese Sesame Sauce

The recover way of eating targets 50 percent of calories contributed by carbohydrates, in particular high-quality carbohydrates, such as whole grains. You may think you're already eating whole grains because, the last time you ordered a turkey sandwich in a restaurant, you remembered to ask the waitress for whole wheat bread. But the kind of "whole grain" you really want to aim for is the original stuff, the unprocessed grain itself, which takes some chewing and has a rich, nutty flavor. Because they contain all of their bran and germ, whole grains provide you with valuable fiber, as well as fat-soluble vitamins and healthy oils. These are truly nourishing foods for recovery.

Okay, perhaps now you get the idea, but you just need some hand-holding when it comes to preparing whole grains. Don't worry—they cook up just like white rice; they just take a little longer. In the following recipes, I've given you a variety of grains to try out, in appealing dishes that may easily become regulars in your kitchen. They feature the familiar grains whole wheat, brown rice, and barley, as well as less common ones, including buckwheat, quinoa, and wild rice.

Grain Cooking Times

Use the quantities and times given in this chart as a general guide for cooking whole grains. They take longer to cook than refined grains do. The grains' official cooking time starts when the liquid that the grains are in has come to a boil. At the end of the cooking time, let the pot stand, covered, for 5 minutes or more, to allow the remaining steam to distribute evenly throughout the grains.

GRAIN COOKING TIMES		
1 CUP GRAIN	COOKING LIQUID	COOKING TIME
BARLEY, PEARLED	3 CUPS	30 MINUTES
BROWN RICE	2½ CUPS	40 MINUTES
COUSCOUS, WHOLE-GRAIN	1½ CUPS	10 MINUTES
KASHA	2 CUPS, BOILING	15 MINUTES
ROLLED OATS, CHEWY TEXTURE	2¼ CUPS	15 MINUTES
OATS, STEEL-CUT	2 CUPS	30 MINUTES
OATS, WHOLE	2 CUPS	55–60 MINUTES
QUINOA	2 CUPS	15 MINUTES
WILD RICE	3 CUPS	30 MINUTES

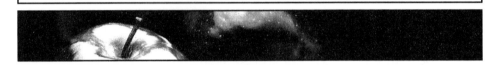

Tabbouleh
(Menu 17)

This Middle Eastern specialty, served at room temperature, is prepared with two fresh herbs, parsley and mint, both of which aid digestion, and is a good choice especially in the early phase of recovery, when this body function may be weak.

YIELD: 6 SERVINGS

1 cup fine- or medium-grind bulgur
2 1/2 cups boiling water
2 ripe tomatoes
1 cup finely chopped fresh parsley, preferably flat-leaf

2 scallions, chopped finely
1/2 cup fresh lemon juice
1 teaspoon salt
1/2 cup extra-virgin olive oil
2 tablespoons finely cut fresh mint

1. Put the bulgur in a bowl and pour the boiling water over it. Stir once and set aside while the grains soak up the liquid. Finely ground bulgur will be tender in 15 to 20 minutes; medium-grind, in 20 to 25 minutes. If there is any remaining water, put the bulgur in a sieve and press down on it.

2. To the bowl of bulgur, add the tomatoes, parsley, scallions, lemon juice, and salt. Toss together gently but thoroughly with a fork.

3. Just before serving, stir in the olive oil and mint. Serve at room temperature or chilled.

Green Bell Peppers Stuffed with Brown Rice and Spices

Brown rice supplies you with a good amount of magnesium for heart and bone health. The addition of sunflower seeds boosts the nutrient content, adding the minerals potassium, iron, zinc, calcium, magnesium, manganese, and copper, plus vitamin B_6 and niacin. Look for opportunities like this one to give a standard recipe a nutrition upgrade.

YIELD: 6 SERVINGS

1^1/$_2$ cups short-grain brown rice
3 cups water
3 tablespoons extra-virgin olive oil
1 medium-size onion, peeled and diced
2 tablespoons sunflower seeds
1^1/$_2$ teaspoons ground cinnamon

1 teaspoon ground allspice
1 large ripe tomato, diced
2 tablespoons dried currants
^{1}/$_2$ teaspoon dried tarragon
2 teaspoons fresh lemon juice
6 medium-size green bell peppers

1. Put the rice and water in a saucepan with a tight-fitting lid. Bring to a boil. Cover and lower the heat to low. Cook until the rice is tender, about 40 minutes

2. Meanwhile, put the olive oil in a skillet and add the onions and sunflower seeds. Sauté over medium heat, stirring occasionally, until the onions become translucent, about 7 minutes.

3. Add the cinnamon and allspice, stirring into the onion mixture, heating the spices to develop their flavor. Add the tomato, currants, tarragon, and lemon juice. Mix well.

4. When the rice has finished cooking, add it to the onion mixture and stir. Set aside.

Preheat the oven to 375°F.

5. Cut the tops off the peppers and reserve. Scoop out the seeds. Fill a large pot with water and bring to a boil. Add the peppers and parboil for 2 minutes. Transfer with tongs to a work surface.

6. Spoon the rice mixture into the peppers. Replace the pepper tops and arrange the peppers in a baking pan filled with ^{1}/$_2$ inch of water, to prevent the peppers from burning on the bottom.

7. Bake the peppers until tender, about 45 minutes, and serve.

Quinoa Pilaf

Quinoa (pronounced keen-wah) is one of the ancient grains, along with amaranth and kamut, worth your attention because of its high nutritional value. It offers more protein than do most grains and also contains more calcium, magnesium, and especially potassium, as well as a range of B vitamins. The tiny grains, actually the fruit of a plant related to beets, have an appealing, grassy, light flavor. Since they are naturally coated with a bitter substance that wards off insects, you need to rinse off quinoa before cooking it. Commercial quinoa has had most of that substance removed, but rinsing it off a couple of times is worth the effort, so no traces can spoil the grain's delicate flavor.

YIELD: 4 SERVINGS
1 cup quinoa
2 tablespoons unrefined safflower oil
$1/2$ medium-size onion, peeled and
    chopped into small bits
1 tablespoon minced fresh parsley
Salt and pepper
$1^3/4$ cups chicken broth, plus extra

1. Rinse the quinoa in a fine-mesh sieve in several changes of water. Set aside.

2. Heat the oil in a deep-sided skillet and add the onions. Cook over medium heat, stirring occasionally, until onion begins to soften, about 5 minutes.

3. Add the quinoa and parsley and cook for at least 5 minutes, stirring as the quinoa absorbs the oil. Season to taste with salt and pepper.

4. Pour the broth into the skillet. Cover and cook for about 15 minutes, until the quinoa is tender. If all the broth has been absorbed before the quinoa has finished cooking, add 3 or 4 more tablespoons of liquid and continue to cook the grain until tender.

Wild Rice Pilaf with Pecans ❧

Wild rice is known for its nutty flavor and satisfyingly chewy texture. As in this pilaf, it's usually mixed with other grains. While not as rich in nutrients as many other grains, it does add a gourmet touch to a health-food standard like brown rice.

YIELD: 6 SERVINGS

1 cup wild rice, rinsed
1 cup short-grain brown rice, rinsed
5 cups chicken broth, vegetable
    broth, or water
1 teaspoon salt
2 tablespoons unrefined safflower oil
1/2 cup pecans
Salt and pepper

2 tablespoons butter or butter
    substitute, such as Smart Balance
    Buttery Spread
1 medium-size onion, peeled and
    chopped finely
1/2 teaspoon dried sage
1/2 teaspoon dried thyme

1. In a medium-size saucepan, put the wild rice, brown rice, broth and salt. Cover and bring to a boil over high heat. Lower the heat to low and cook undisturbed for 40 minutes. The rice is done when the grains have puffed up and are quite tender. If the rice is not done, continue to cook, adding more liquid if necessary.

2. Meanwhile, in a sauté pan, heat the oil and add the pecans. Roast the pecans over medium heat, stirring, until they begin to smell fragrant and are lightly browned, about 10 minutes. Season with salt and pepper. Transfer to a small bowl and set aside.

3. Using the same sauté pan, melt the butter and add the onion, sage, and thyme. Cook over medium heat, stirring occasionally, for about 10 minutes.

4. When the rice is cooked, fluff with a fork to separate the grains. Add the onion mixture and toss to combine.

5. Transfer the pilaf to a serving bowl and top with the roasted pecans. Serve immediately.

Breakfast Polenta ♨
(Menu 4)

This breakfast combo also makes a nourishing light lunch.

YIELD: 4 SERVINGS

1 (16-ounce) tube precooked polenta
2 eggs
1 cup bread crumbs, preferably whole wheat

3 tablespoons extra-virgin olive oil
$^1/_2$ cantaloupe, sliced
8 slices prosciutto

1. Cut the polenta crosswise in $^1/_2$-inch-thick slices. Crack the eggs into a bowl and beat. Cover a plate with the bread crumbs. Dip each polenta slice into the eggs and then the bread crumbs.

2. Heat the oil in a large skillet over medium heat. Cook the polenta until lightly browned on both sides. Serve with melon and prosciutto.

Barley Scented
with Summer Savory ♨

For variety, remember to have some barley. It's loaded with soluble fiber for cleansing and good digestion, and has a nice chewy texture. Pearled barley is the standard kind you'll find in supermarkets but it's not strictly a whole grain; that's unhulled barley, which is sold in health food stores. The unhulled kind provides even more nutrients but takes more than twice as long to cook and is very, very chewy. Start with pearled barley for ease; once you're feeling more adventurous, you can try your hand with the unhulled variety.

YIELD: 4 SERVINGS

2 tablespoons butter substitute, such as Smart Balance Buttery Spread
$^1/_2$ cup chopped onion or shallots
1 cup pearled barley, rinsed

$2^1/_2$ cups chicken or vegetable broth
1 teaspoon dried summer savory
Salt and pepper

1. Melt the butter substitute in a skillet set over medium heat. Add the onions and cook, stirring occasionally, until they become translucent and soften, about 5 minutes.

2. Add the barley to the onions and cook, stirring, for 1 minute. Add the broth and summer savory. Season with salt and pepper. Bring to a boil.

3. Reduce the heat to low. Cover the skillet and cook the barley for 30 minutes, until all the liquid is absorbed. (Add additional liquid by the tablespoonful and cook a little longer if all the liquid has been absorbed and the barley is not quite soft enough for your taste.) Adjust the seasonings and serve.

Mexican Rice
(Menu 19)

Although this dish is usually made with white rice, the assertive flavors of the other ingredients taste just right with the fuller nuttiness of brown rice. Cooking the rice in the savory sauce before steaming it permeates the grain with flavor.

YIELD: 4 SERVINGS
1 medium-size tomato, seeded, or
   $1/2$ cup canned tomatoes
1 small wedge onion
1 clove garlic
3 tablespoons unrefined safflower oil
1 cup brown rice
2 cups chicken broth or water
Salt and pepper

1. Trim and chop the tomato and onion.

2. Put the tomato, onion, and garlic in a food processor and puree.

3. Heat the oil in a medium-size pot and add the rice. Cook, stirring occasionally, until the rice turns a pale golden color, about 10 minutes. Tip the pan to drain away any excess oil.

4. Add the tomato mixture to the rice and cook over high heat, stirring constantly, until the mixture is almost dry, about 3 minutes.

5. Stir the chicken broth into the rice and cook, covered, for 40 to 50 minutes, or until the rice is tender. Toss with a fork. Season with salt and pepper, and serve.

Kasha with Mushrooms and Walnuts

The earthy flavor of kasha (also called buckwheat groats) makes for a satis-fying, chilly-weather dish, when paired with autumn ingredients such as mushrooms and walnuts. Kasha is dry roasted; it is not rinsed before cook-ing and is ready in about 10 minutes. Remembering to feed yourself nour-ishing food isn't hard when you have this deliciously satisfying dish on hand.

YIELD: 4 SERVINGS

8 ounces mixed mushrooms, such as shiitake, portobello, cremini, and oyster

2 tablespoons butter substitute, such as Smart Balance Buttery Spread

1 onion, peeled and chopped finely

$1/3$ cup walnuts, chopped coarsely

1 cup kasha

$1/2$ teaspoon dried thyme

$1/2$ teaspoon salt

2 cups chicken broth or water

1. Trim mushrooms and rinse only briefly, as they easily absorb water. Chop coarsely.

2. Heat the butter substitute in a skillet and add the mushrooms and onion. Cover and cook over medium heat until the onions are translucent, about 5 minutes, stirring occasionally.

3. Add the walnuts, stir, and cook, covered, for another 5 minutes. Set aside.

4. Put the kasha, thyme, salt, and broth in a medium-size pot. Cover and bring to a boil. Lower the heat and simmer for 15 minutes, or until all the liquid is absorbed. Turn off the heat.

5. Use a fork to fluff and separate the cooked grains. Add the mushroom mixture and stir to incorporate. Serve with roasted chicken.

Pasta Primavera with Pesto 🍲
(Menu 6)

This recipe is a delicious way to meet Goal 2 of the recovery program, which aims at eating more vegetables.

YIELD: 4 SERVINGS

$1/2$ pound sweet red bell peppers
$1/2$ pound broccoli
$1/2$ pound cherry tomatoes
$1/2$ pound mushrooms
1 clove garlic
$1/4$ cup extra-virgin olive oil

Salt
12 ounces spaghetti (see Note)
6 tablespoons bottled basil pesto, or to taste
Parmesan cheese (optional)

1. Cut the peppers and any broccoli stems into narrow slices, chop the remaining broccoli head into bite-size pieces, and halve the cherry tomatoes and mushrooms. Mince the garlic.

2. Put the olive oil, vegetables, and garlic in a large skillet and cook over medium heat, stirring occasionally, until tender, about 15 minutes.

3. Meanwhile, fill a pot with water, add a pinch of salt, and bring to a rolling boil. Add the spaghetti and cook according to the package instructions, about 12 minutes. Drain in a colander and return to the pot. Heat for 30 seconds to evaporate any remaining liquid.

4. Add the pesto and toss the pasta to coat. Divide among four individual bowls. Top with the vegetables and serve. Add grated Parmesan cheese, if desired.

Note: To upgrade the pasta to a whole grain, try DeBoles, De Cecco, and Eden brands. You can also sample Eden's 50/50 line of pastas, made with half white flour and half whole wheat.

Storing Whole Grains

Whole grains require special care in storing. Unlike refined grains, they still retain their germ, an oily component that can go rancid fairly quickly. Besides tasting stale, rancid grain has oxidized, generating free radicals that, once consumed, can damage cells—just what a body in recovery doesn't need.

Stored in containers with screw-on lids, in a cool, dry place, whole grains and cereals keep fresh for at least six months. Keep whole-grain flours and mixes refrigerated or frozen. Refrigerated, they'll keep for about four months; frozen, for one year.

Another freshness strategy is to buy stone-ground grains. Grinding the grain with stones keeps the germ from being heated and retains the freshness of the oil in the germ. Such grains still need to be stored in airtight containers in a cold place.

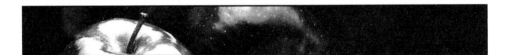

Angel Hair Pasta with Clam Sauce
(Menu 11)

Stick to recovery eating and please family and friends with this mouthwatering, time-honored Italian pasta classic.

YIELD: 4 SERVINGS

2 (6.5-ounce) cans chopped clams
3 tablespoons extra-virgin olive oil
3 cloves garlic, minced
3 tablespoons fresh parsley, chopped finely

1 teaspoon mixed Italian dried herbs
Pinch of hot pepper flakes
$1/2$ cup chicken broth
1 tablespoon lemon juice
6 ounces angel hair pasta

1. Pour the chopped clams and juice into a sieve set over a bowl and reserve the clam juice. Set aside the clams.

2. Heat the olive oil in a large skillet over medium heat. Add the garlic and cook for about 30 seconds. Add the parsley, dried herbs, and pepper flakes, and stir

to combine. Add the reserved clam juice, chicken broth, and lemon juice. Simmer for 3 to 4 minutes. Season with salt, cover, remove from the heat, and set aside.

3. Meanwhile, bring a large pot of salted water to a rolling boil. Cook the pasta for 6 to 7 minutes, or according to package instructions. Drain the pasta and add to the clam juice mixture. Add the reserved clams.

4. Cook the pasta and sauce over medium-low heat, tossing constantly, until all the sauce is absorbed, about 3 minutes. Serve immediately with Italian-Style Spinach (see page 206) and Parmesan cheese.

Pasta with Fresh Peas and Prosciutto

Peas, normally thought of as a vegetable, are actually a legume and a good source of protein.

YIELD: 4 SERVINGS
1 pound fresh peas (unshelled weight)
$1/4$ pound sliced prosciutto, cut into
     strips
1 pound pasta, preferably made with
     spelt flour
$1/2$ cup low-fat ricotta cheese
Parmesan cheese
Pepper

1. Shell the peas and cook in a small amount of boiling water for 5 to 10 minutes (depending on size of peas), until tender. Add the prosciutto and cook for an additional minute. Set aside.

2. Bring a pot of salted water to a rolling boil. Add the pasta and cook according to the package instructions. When the pasta is cooked to your desired degree of doneness, drain the pasta and return it to its cooking pot. Heat for 30 seconds to evaporate any remaining liquid.

3. Briefly reheat the peas and prosciutto. Using a slotted spoon, transfer to a large serving bowl. Add the ricotta and cooked pasta, and toss to combine. Add Parmesan cheese and pepper, and toss again. Serve immediately.

Buckwheat Soba Noodles in Chinese Sesame Sauce

This sauce is a winner, a mix of sweet and savory, with a richness contributed by the sesame paste. Buckwheat is not wheat at all but the triangular seeds of an herb; but be aware, if you're wheat sensitive, soba noodles also contain some actual wheat.

YIELD: 4 SERVINGS

^{1}/$_4$ cup soy sauce
^{1}/$_4$ cup plus 2 tablespoons sesame
   paste
3 tablespoons rice vinegar
2 tablespoons honey
2 cloves garlic, peeled and chopped
2 sprigs cilantro, leaves only, chopped
Dash of Tabasco sauce, or to taste
1 (8-ounce) package soba noodles
2 scallions, chopped
^{1}/$_4$ cup roasted peanuts

1. Place the soy sauce, sesame paste, vinegar, honey, garlic, cilantro, and Tabasco in a food processor fitted with a metal blade. Process until thoroughly combined.

   (If you wish to mix the sauce manually, the garlic and cilantro should be minced in advance; then, using a whisk, first mix together the soy sauce, sesame paste, and vinegar before adding the other sauce ingredients.) Set the sauce aside.

2. Fill a pot with water, bring to a boil, and cook the noodles according to the package instructions.

3. Transfer the noodles to a serving bowl. Spoon the sauce over the noodles and toss to combine. Garnish with the scallions and peanuts. Serve at room temperature or refrigerate for 1 hour to serve chilled.

Beans and Other Legumes

The Recipes:

Pinto Beans with a Mexican Accent
Molasses-Sweetened Baked Beans
Lentils with Caramelized Onions ✍
North African Chickpea and Tomato Soup
Black-Eyed Peas and Greens
Soybean Succotash
Italian-Style White Bean and Vegetable Soup ✍
Three-Bean Salad
Arugula Salad with Chickpeas, Artichokes,
and Roasted Sweet Red Peppers
Black Bean Pâté

If the only beans you eat are canned baked beans, here's your chance to expand your bean repertoire. The following recipes feature a variety of legumes, beans being only one kind. Peas and lentils are also part of this food family. They all benefit recovery, thanks to their fiber content and the many nutrients they offer, including calcium, magnesium, potassium, and zinc, as well as small amounts of the B vitamins. Legumes are also a source of low-fat protein.

Dried peas and lentils cook up quickly but dried beans take longer, a real stopper for many cooks and one reason they are rarely prepared from scratch in most kitchens. This is a true culinary loss because, when cooked, dried beans take the prize for flavor and texture. Bottled beans come in second, and canned beans last. But preparing dried beans isn't as complicated as you may expect. First, you don't have to bother soaking them the night before to shorten their cooking time. This only saves you 15 to 30 minutes. It's easier to just get a head start the day you're preparing the beans. Cook them in a pot of water as you cook something else or answer your e-mail, and most kinds will be tender in an hour or a little longer.

If the darn things just won't soften up, you probably started with stale dried beans, not fresh dried beans. Here are some remedies.

▸ Buy beans from a store that sells a lot of them, to avoid bringing home beans that have been sitting on the shelves for months.

▸ Don't buy beans that are faded, dry looking, and wrinkled—all signs that they are of a certain age.

▸ Toss out beans that have been sitting around your kitchen for eons, and repurchase them. The best time to stock up is in the fall, just after the yearly bean harvest.

You may be wary of beans because of their notoriety for giving people digestive gas; if you have only consumed beans occasionally, you may have had firsthand experience with this. However, simply eating beans more frequently will increase your body's tolerance for them. You can also draw out some of the bean sugars that cause gas by putting the beans in a pot filled with 3 quarts of water and bringing this to a boil. Then cool the pot and refrigerate the beans overnight. Drain the soaking water, rinse the beans and proceed as usual with your recipe, using fresh water. Or alternatively, take advantage of Beano, a commercially sold product found in grocery stores, which supplies the enzymes that go to work breaking up the offending sugars. When eating beans, take some Beano with your first bite, 1 Beano tablet or 5 drops of Beano liquid for each $1/2$-cup serving.

Pinto Beans with a Mexican Accent

When shopping for oregano, look for Mexican oregano, which is especially aromatic. Alternatively, cook these beans with epazote, a pungent wild herb found in Latin markets, which is traditionally cooked with beans. Epazote, which has an earthy flavor, is considered medicinal, reducing gas.

YIELD: 4 SERVINGS
1 pound pinto beans, washed and
   picked over
2 cloves garlic, crushed and peeled
2 bay leaves
1 teaspoon dried oregano
2 teaspoons salt

1. Put the beans in a large pot filled with enough water to cover the beans. Add the garlic, bay leaves, and dried oregano. Over high heat, bring the water to a boil. If necessary, skim away any foam that accumulates on top of the water. Lower the heat to medium or medium-low so that the beans simmer. Partially cover the pot.

2. Cook the beans, stirring occasionally with a wooden spoon. When the beans start to become tender, add the salt. Using salt at this point in the cooking process will not cause the beans to toughen.

3. Continue to cook the beans, gently stirring from time to time until they reach your desired degree of tenderness. If necessary, add additional water.

4. Drain in a colander set in a bowl, to catch the cooking juices. Serve as is or use in another recipe. Another option is to freeze any unused beans. Beans freeze very successfully, retaining their original texture and flavor. They're a great alternative when you want beans quickly but don't want the kind that comes in a can. Frozen airtight in their cooking liquid, they're good for 3 months.

Molasses–Sweetened Baked Beans

Blackstrap molasses, richer in minerals than milder-tasting lighter grades, delivers calcium, iron, and potassium. Refined sugar, the usual sweetener for baked beans, supplies no minerals at all.

YIELD: 6 CUPS

2 cups dried kidney beans, sorted
  and washed
1 onion, trimmed and diced
1/4 cup blackstrap molasses,
  preferably unsulfured

2 tablespoons unrefined safflower oil
1 tablespoon cider vinegar
1 1/2 teaspoons dried mustard
1 teaspoon salt

Preheat the oven to 325°F.

1. In an ovenproof casserole, combine the beans, onion, molasses, safflower oil, cider vinegar, and mustard, and stir. Add 5 cups of water and stir again.

2. Cover casserole and bake for 8 hours.

3. Remove from the oven and, before serving, stir in the salt.

Lentils with Caramelized Onions 🍂

Lentils are an excellent source of folate, a nutrient that repairs DNA, helping stop the spread of cancer.

YIELD: 4 SERVINGS

2 cups green or brown lentils
1 stalk celery, halved
1 clove garlic
1 bay leaf
Pinch of dried thyme
1 medium-size onion
2 tablespoons extra-virgin olive oil

1. Rinse and sort through the lentils for pebbles and other foreign matter. Fill a pot with water, bring to a boil, and add the lentils along with the celery,

garlic, bay leaf, and thyme. Cook, uncovered, over medium heat until the lentils are tender, about 45 minutes. Drain the lentils and remove the celery, garlic, and bay leaf.

2. Meanwhile, peel the onion and slice crosswise into very thin slices. Using a large skillet, heat the olive oil and add the onions. Cook over medium heat, stirring occasionally, for 10 to 15 minutes, until the onions begin to turn a rich golden color, a sign they are caramelizing and becoming sweeter.

3. Add the onions to the cooked lentils. Reheat the lentil mixture briefly, if necessary. Serve as an accompaniment to chops or paired with a grain dish to create a vegetarian meal.

North African Chickpea and Tomato Soup

Chickpeas are good for recovery, supplying calcium for the bones and vitamin A to maintain the lining of the digestive tract. If you're not accustomed to eating beans and they don't appeal to you, this soup is a good way to start. In this recipe, the chickpeas disappear into a tomato soup accented with fragrant spices. The chickpeas also thicken the soup, giving it a hearty texture.

YIELD: 2 GENEROUS LUNCH PORTIONS

1/2 yellow onion
2 tablespoons extra-virgin olive oil
3 cups prepared tomato soup, such as Trader Joe's boxed Organic Creamy Tomato Soup

1 (15-ounce) can chickpeas, drained
1/4 teaspoon ground cinnamon
1/4 teaspoon ground ginger
1/4 teaspoon ground turmeric
Salt and pepper

1. Peel and slice the onion. Heat the olive oil in a skillet and add the onions. Cook over medium heat until the onion softens and turns golden, 5 to 7 minutes.

2. Put the onion in a food processor or blender. Add the tomato soup, chickpeas, cinnamon, ginger, and turmeric. Process until thoroughly combined. Season with salt and pepper.

3. Transfer the soup to a pot and cook over medium heat for 10 minutes to develop the flavors. To round out the meal, serve with whole wheat pita bread, goat or feta cheese, radishes, scallions, and marinated black olives.

Be an Expert Bean Counter

Figuring out how many beans to cook can leave you guessing. Here are some guidelines.

▶ Beans double or triple their bulk during cooking.
▶ The size of a side serving of cooked beans is ¹/₂ to 1 cup.
▶ You'll need about 1 to 1¹/₂ cups of cooked beans for a main course.

To get you started cooking beans, try my first recipe for Pinto Beans with a Mexican Accent. The steps take you through the basic procedure that also applies to cooking other sorts of beans.

Black-Eyed Peas and Greens

Black-eyed peas, a staple in Southern cooking, are the backdrop for the down-home flavors of ham hocks, collard greens, and hot sauce. Have this hearty combination of ingredients as a side dish or call it dinner.

YIELD: 6 SERVINGS

2 cups black-eyed peas, washed and picked over
2 smoked ham hocks
1 large onion, peeled and chopped

1 small bunch collard greens or kale, trimmed and chopped
Pepper
Hot sauce
Vinegar

1. Put the black-eyed peas in a large pot with enough water to cover the beans. Bring to a boil over high heat, skimming away any foam, if necessary.

2. Add the ham hocks, onion, and greens. Season with pepper. Lower the heat to medium or medium-low, so the bean mixture simmers. Partially cover the pot and cook for about an hour. Stir once or twice, using a wooden spoon. The beans should become very tender.

3. Remove the pot from the heat. Use tongs to transfer the ham hocks to a work surface. Trim the meat from the bones and chop the meat. Add the meat to the bean mixture and season with salt. Serve as is or add hot sauce and/or vinegar to taste.

Soybean Succotash

According to research, alcohol abuse elevates estrogen levels in pre-menopausal women. Phytoestrogens to the rescue—those compounds in plant foods that help restore normal hormone levels. A prime source of phytoestrogens is soybeans, high in certain phytoestrogens that are especially powerful. Here's a good reason to update that classic American dish, succotash, and replace the usual lima beans with soy.

YIELD: 6 SERVINGS

2 cups frozen soybeans (also called edamame)
1 green bell pepper
1 scallion
1 tablespoon unrefined safflower oil

1 (10-ounce) package frozen corn
1/4 teaspoon paprika
1/2 cup milk
1 teaspoon butter
Salt and pepper

1. Put the soybeans in a medium-size pot and cover with water. Cook over medium-high heat until the soybeans soften, about 10 minutes. Drain and transfer soybeans to a large bowl. Set aside.

2. Core the pepper, remove the seeds, and dice. Trim the scallion and cut crosswise into small bits.

3. In the pot used to cook the soybeans, put the oil, pepper, and scallion. Cook over medium heat, stirring frequently, until the vegetables soften, about 7 minutes.

4. Add the cooked soybeans, corn, and paprika, and simmer until the corn is tender, about 10 minutes.

5. Add the milk and butter and raise the heat to medium-high. Cook, uncovered, until liquid reduces somewhat, about 3 minutes. Season with salt and pepper, and serve.

Italian-Style White Bean and Vegetable Soup 🥬

This hearty soup makes a complete meal when coupled with whole-grain bread.

YIELD: 4 SERVINGS

3 tablespoons extra-virgin olive oil
2 carrots, peeled and sliced
2 medium-size onions, peeled and sliced
2 stalks celery, trimmed and sliced
1 fennel bulb, trimmed and chopped
2 cloves garlic, peeled and crushed

1 (15-ounce) can white beans
1 (15-ounce) can chopped tomatoes
2 zucchini, trimmed and sliced thinly
1 quart chicken or vegetable broth
2 tablespoons bottled pesto
Salt and pepper

1. Using a large pot, heat the olive oil. Add the carrots, onions, celery, fennel, and garlic. Lower the heat to medium and sauté the vegetables until the onions begin to brown slightly, stirring occasionally, 7 to 10 minutes.

2. Add the beans, tomatoes, zucchini, and broth. Stir in the pesto.

3. Raise the heat to medium-high and bring the soup to a boil. Lower the heat, cover, and simmer for 30 minutes, until the vegetables are tender. Season with salt and pepper.

Three-Bean Salad
(Menu 7)

When you're in the mood for deli flavors, have some of this bean salad, which gives you protein and fiber, a healthier choice than potato salad that is heavy on carbs.

YIELD: 6 SERVINGS

1/2 pound fresh green beans, or 1 (15-ounce) can
1 (15-ounce) can kidney beans, drained and rinsed
1 (15-ounce can) chickpeas, drained and rinsed

1 stalk celery
1/4 red onion
1/3 cup Basic Vinaigrette with Flaxseed Oil (page 268)

1. Cut off and discard the stem end of the green beans and cut into 1-inch lengths. In a small pot, bring $1/2$ cup water to a boil, add the beans, and steam until bright green, about 4 minutes. Using a slotted spoon, transfer the green beans to a large bowl.

2. Dice the celery and finely chop the onion.

3. Add the celery and onion, along with the canned beans, to the green beans.

4. Add the dressing and toss the ingredients. Let marinate for at least 1 hour or overnight, to develop the flavors.

Arugula Salad with Chickpeas, Artichokes, and Roasted Sweet Red Peppers

Expand your lettuce vocabulary to arugula, a somewhat bitter, dark salad green. It's a rich source of iron, vitamin A, and vitamin C. This recipe also features homemade broiled sweet red peppers for richer flavor than the commercial kind. But if you're short on time, substitute bottled peppers for fresh, rather than miss out on this healthy gourmet recipe.

YIELD: 4 SERVINGS

1 sweet red pepper, or 4 large pieces bottled, roasted red peppers
$1/2$ pound arugula
2 cups chickpeas, canned or preferably bottled

1 (12-ounce) jar marinated artichokes, drained
$1/4$ cup extra-virgin olive oil
2 tablespoons lemon juice
Salt and pepper

1. To skin the fresh pepper, pierce the pepper with a long-handled fork or hold with tongs. On a gas stove, ignite one of the burners and hold the pepper directly over the flame. Turn the pepper after an area of the skin has charred, every 1 to 2 minutes. To loosen the skin, when all sides of the pepper have blackened, put the pepper in a covered bowl, or in a paper bag and then close the bag. Set aside for at least 10 minutes.

2. Meanwhile, put the arugula, chickpeas, and artichokes into a large bowl.

(recipe continues, next page)

3. Peel the pepper, remove the core and seeds, and cut into bite-size pieces. Add to the arugula salad. Toss all the ingredients to combine.

4. To make the dressing, in a small bowl, mix together the olive oil and lemon juice and season with salt and pepper, or use Anchovy Vinaigrette (see page 270). Drizzle the dressing over the salad and toss to thoroughly coat. Serve this salad as a main course for lunch or as a side salad with pasta.

Black Bean Pâté

Instead of pork fat and its saturated fat, this pâté takes its richness from pureed black beans.

YIELD: 1 LOAF

4–5 cups soaked black beans (from 2 cups dried), or 3 (15-ounce) cans black beans, drained
1 stalk celery, trimmed and chopped coarsely
1 carrot, chopped coarsely
2 bay leaves
2 tablespoons extra-virgin olive oil

2 medium-size onions, peeled and sliced
2 teaspoons dried thyme
2 teaspoons salt
1/4 teaspoon black pepper
3 cloves garlic peeled and chopped
1 cup whole wheat bread crumbs

1. If using soaked beans, put the beans in a large pot and add 4 cups of water to cover. Add the celery, carrot, and bay leaves. Cover the pot and, over high heat, bring to a boil. Lower the heat to low and simmer for 1 hour, until the beans are soft. Drain the beans and discard the bay leaves. Set aside.

2. In a large skillet, heat the oil and add the onions, thyme, salt, and pepper. Stir to combine. Cook over medium heat for 5 minutes. Add the garlic, cover, and lower the heat to low, cooking an additional 10 minutes, until the onions are very soft. Add the cooked beans, or the canned beans, and stir well. Remove from the heat.

Preheat the oven to 350°F.

3. Put the bean mixture in a food processor or blender and puree, adding the celery and carrots in batches. Transfer each batch to a bowl as you proceed.

4. Stir 3/4 cup of bread crumbs into the pureed bean mixture. (If using a blender, it may be necessary to add some additional liquid to thin the bean mixture so it's easier to puree. Also add an additional 1/4 cup of bread crumbs.)

5. Oil the side and bottom of a 4-cup loaf pan. Dust with the remaining ¼ cup of bread crumbs. Spoon the pâté into the loaf pan and smooth the surface of the pâté with the back of a wet spoon. Bake 30 minutes, until the pâté begins to pull away from the sides of the pan. Remove from the oven.

6. Let the pâté cool for at least 20 minutes before removing from the pan. Slip a knife around the sides of the loaf. Place a plate on top and, holding both the pan and the plate, quickly flip the two over. Lift up loaf pan and serve pâté as an appetizer, garnished with parsley and radishes, or sliced as a luncheon entrée with a side of salad.

Vegetables

The Recipes:

Carrots with Their Tops, Mediterranean-Style 🥬
Green Beans with Shallots 🥬
Baked Beets 🥬
Braised Leeks
Cabbage-Tomato Gratin
Down-South Okra
Sautéed Brussels Sprouts
Steamed Artichoke with Herbs and Garlic
Winter Squash in Coconut Milk 🥬
Stir-Fried Broccoli and Shiitake Mushrooms
Italian-Style Spinach
Pan-Fried Tomatoes
Sautéed Kale
Sautéed Sweet Red Peppers
Greek-Style Green Beans
Oven-Baked "Fries"
Boiled Potatoes 🥬
Baked Sweet Potatoes 🥬

One of the goals of the second phase of the recovery diet is to eat a greater variety of foods and here's your chance—by preparing some of the following vegetable recipes. Many people consider they are eating an assortment of veggies when they go beyond carrots, tomatoes, broccoli, and peas, and have some mushrooms. The recipes include these familiar ingredients, but some may also take you into new territory. When is the last time you had okra, celery root, leeks, or artichokes, not to mention fresh-cooked beets or winter squash? If what's been stopping you from cooking these less common vegetables is that you simply don't know how to approach them, have no fear. The following recipes for these foods start with the basics of trimming, slicing, and readying them for easy cooking.

Each of these vegetables also offers its own particular benefits for recovery. Some are a source of fiber for cleansing, whereas others supply you with special vitamins and minerals to replenish deficiencies and repair your body. You'll also be glad for their more immediate rewards: delectable and intriguing flavors and textures that can turn an everyday meal into a special treat.

Carrots with Their Tops, Mediterranean-Style 🥕

Carrots are an abundant source of the antioxidant beta-carotene, the plant form of vitamin A.

YIELD: 4 SERVINGS
1 bunch carrots, with tops
¹/₂ lemon, sliced crosswise
3 cloves garlic, crushed and peeled
2 tablespoons extra-virgin olive oil
8 brine-cured black olives, such as
    kalamata
Salt and pepper

Preheat the oven to 400°F.

1. Trim the tops from the carrots. Reserve a few sprigs and chop enough to produce 1 tablespoon of finely chopped tops. Rinse and peel the carrots. Cut in half lengthwise and then crosswise into thirds.

2. In a shallow baking dish, mix together the carrots, carrot tops, lemon, garlic, and oil.

3. Put the carrots in the preheated oven and bake, stirring from time to time, until tender and lightly browned, about 45 minutes. Add the olives and bake for an additional 10 minutes. Season with salt and pepper. Serve.

Green Beans with Shallots ⍒

Green beans are an excellent source of fiber, which helps ensure normal function of the digestive tract.

YIELD: 4 SERVINGS
1 pound green beans
1 tablespoon unrefined safflower oil
1 teaspoon butter
2 shallots, peeled and chopped finely
Salt and pepper

1. Trim and discard the stem end of the beans but not the tapered blossom end. Bring a pot of salted water to a boil. Drop the beans into the water and cook until tender but still bright green, about 8 minutes.

2. Put the oil and butter in a large skillet set over medium-high heat and add the shallots. Cook for 1 minute, stirring frequently. Add the green beans. Lower the heat and sauté the vegetables, stirring occasionally, for 5 minutes. Season with salt and pepper, and serve.

Baked Beets ⍒

Beets do their part in reducing fatty infiltration of the liver, thanks to betaine, a phytonutrient they contain, but they can be messy to prepare if you don't know the easy way to fix them. Baking the beets is the answer, reducing the chance of getting their staining juices all over you. Baking also retains more beet flavor. Try the handy procedure in the following recipe. (To make sure all the beets are done cooking about the same time, start with beets that are about the same size.)

YIELD: 6 SERVINGS
8 medium-size or 4 large beets, about
    1 1/2–2 pounds
2 tablespoons unrefined safflower oil
    or butter
Salt and pepper
Garnish of chopped fresh parsley,
    lemon juice, or orange zest

Preheat the oven to 400°F.

1. Thoroughly wash the beets. Wrap each individually in aluminum foil. Place in a roasting pan.

2. Bake the beets for 45 minutes to 1¹/₂ hours, depending on their size. Beets are done cooking when a thin-bladed knife is able to pierce one with little resistance.

3. To serve immediately, unwrap each beet and secure with a fork as you remove the peel with a knife. To reserve beets for another meal, cook, refrigerate in their foil wrap, and then peel when ready to use. To reheat the beets, slice or cut into wedges and cook in oil or butter.

4. Season with salt and pepper, and garnish with parsley and lemon juice or orange zest.

Braised Leeks

Like other members of the onion family, leeks help fight inflammation. Remember leeks when you're trying to think of a side dish, to add their delicate, gourmet flavor to meats and poultry main courses. The only challenge in cooking leeks is to be sure to wash them thoroughly, as their leaves almost always contain a great deal of sand.

YIELD: 4 SERVINGS
4 leeks
2 tablespoons butter
Salt and pepper
¹/₂ cup chicken or vegetable broth
1 teaspoon chopped fresh parsley
1 tablespoon freshly squeezed lemon
   juice

1. To trim and wash the leeks, first remove the tough green leaves. Then cut off the root end, slice the leeks lengthwise in half, almost to the root end, and finally, spread out the leaves. Hold the leeks under running water and spread the cut layers, fanning them like a hand of cards. Now fill a large bowl with water and slosh the root end of the leeks up and down to allow any remaining sand to drop to the bottom. Cut the leeks into 4-inch-long sections.

(recipe continues, next page)

2. Using a skillet large enough to fit the leeks in a single layer, melt the butter over medium heat. Add the leeks and season with salt and pepper. Cook for 5 minutes, turning the leeks once or twice.

3. Add the broth and parsley. Raise the heat and bring to a boil. Lower the heat, cover, and cook until the leeks are tender, about 20 minutes.

4. Uncover the skillet and, if the leeks are sitting in lots of liquid, raise the heat to boil some away, still making sure the leeks remain moist.

5. Drizzle lemon juice over the leeks. Serve hot, cold, or at room temperature.

Cabbage–Tomato Gratin

Cabbage supplies phytonutrients that play an important role in how the liver detoxifies harmful chemicals and pollutants.

YIELD: 6 SERVINGS

1^1/$_2$ pounds green cabbage
5 tablespoons extra-virgin olive oil
1 (14.5-ounce) can Italian-style
    tomatoes
1 clove garlic, finely chopped

^{1}/$_2$ teaspoon dried basil
Salt and pepper
^{1}/$_4$ cup Italian-seasoned bread
    crumbs, preferably whole wheat

Preheat the oven to 350°F.

1. Using a sharp knife on a cutting board or a food processor fitted with a shredding blade, finely shred the cabbage.

2. Heat 2 tablespoons of water and 3 tablespoons of the olive oil in a large skillet and add the cabbage. Cook over medium heat, covered, stirring occasionally, for 10 minutes, until the cabbage begins to release some juices.

3. Add the tomatoes and their juice, and the garlic and basil, and stir to combine. Season with salt and pepper. Cook, uncovered, for an additional 10 minutes.

4. Transfer the cabbage mixture and juices to an ovenproof dish. Level the top surface of the vegetables and cover with a single layer of tomato slices. Sprinkle bread crumbs over the tomatoes. Drizzle the bread crumbs with the remaining 2 tablespoons of oil. Bake for 1 hour. Serve immediately.

Down-South Okra

Okra is an excellent source of soluble fiber, the part of the vegetable that makes it feel slippery on the tongue. This same fiber stimulates the flow of bile, a cleansing action and an important factor in restoring health in recovery.

YIELD: 4 SERVINGS

1 tablespoon extra-virgin olive oil
1 medium-size onion, peeled and
    chopped
1 stalk celery, chopped finely
1 medium-size green bell pepper,
    seeded and chopped finely

1 tablespoon tomato paste
$1/4$ teaspoon cayenne, or to taste
1 pound okra, trimmed
Salt

1. Heat the oil in a large skillet over medium-high heat. Add the onion and sauté for 5 minutes, stirring frequently. Add the celery, bell pepper, tomato paste, and cayenne. Cook for 2 minutes.

2. Add 1 cup of water and the okra. Cover, lower the heat, and simmer for 20 minutes, or until the okra is tender but not overly soft. Season with salt.

Sautéed Brussels Sprouts

Like broccoli and cauliflower, Brussels sprouts are a member of the cabbage family of vegetables and have cancer-fighting properties. In a study conducted in the Netherlands, high intake of cruciferous vegetables such as Brussels sprouts was linked to a decreased risk of cancer of the GI tract. Savor these helpful miniature cabbages accented with the woodsy flavor of nutmeg.

YIELD: 4 SERVINGS

$1-1^1/2$ pounds Brussels sprouts,
    trimmed and halved
2 tablespoons unrefined safflower oil
2 tablespoons bread crumbs
$1/8$ teaspoon grated nutmeg
1 tablespoon lemon juice
Salt and pepper

(recipe continues, next page)

1. Over high heat, bring a large pot of water to a boil. Add salt and the Brussels sprouts. Boil the vegetables for 15 minutes, or until tender. Strain the Brussels sprouts, using a colander set in the sink, and rinse briefly in cold water.

2. Put the safflower oil in a large skillet over medium heat. Add the vegetables, bread crumbs, and nutmeg.

3. Reheat the Brussels sprouts and cook for 5 minutes, stirring occasionally. Sprinkle lemon juice over the vegetables and toss. Season with salt and pepper, and serve.

Steamed Artichokes with Herbs and Garlic

Artichokes deserve to be eaten regularly for the many benefits they offer. They stimulate the kidneys and help clear out toxic compounds produced in the gut. They are also a source of B vitamins and fiber.

YIELD: 4 SERVINGS

4 large artichokes
$1/2$ medium-size onion, chopped finely
$1/4$ cup extra-virgin olive oil

2 cloves garlic, peeled and minced
2 sprigs parsley, stems removed and leaves chopped
$1/2$ teaspoon dried basil

1. To prep the artichokes, slice off the stems and tear off and discard the top two or three layers of tough outer leaves.

2. Open and expose the inner leaves and "choke." Remove any thorny leaves. Using a spoon, scoop out and discard the fuzzy matter from the choke.

3. Put 4 cups of water, the onion, oil, garlic, parsley, and basil in a large pot and stir to combine. Place the artichokes in the pot, stem side down. Cover with a tight-fitting lid.

4. Over medium heat, steam the artichokes for 45 minutes to 1 hour. Add additional water if necessary. Artichokes are done cooking when one of the bottom leaves can be easily removed by pulling on it and when the artichoke flesh is tender.

Winter Squash in Coconut Milk 🌀

The type of saturated fat in coconut milk, according to a Finnish study, has only a minimal effect on raising triglycerides and cholesterol. The pear is a source of soluble fiber.

YIELD: 6 SERVINGS

2 pounds winter squash, such as
   Hubbard
1 pear
1 cup light coconut milk
1 (1-inch-long) piece fresh ginger,
   peeled and grated
Salt and pepper

1. Using a very large knife or cleaver, split the squash in half. Peel the skin with a paring knife or vegetable peeler. Remove the seeds and cut the squash into bite-size chunks. Trim the pear, core, and dice.

2. Set a collapsible metal steamer in a large pot filled with about 1 inch of salted water. Place the squash in the steamer. Cover and cook the squash until it is very tender, about 20 minutes.

3. Transfer to a skillet set over medium heat. Add the coconut milk, diced pear, and grated ginger. Stir with a large spoon and cook for about 5 minutes to combine flavors. Season with salt and pepper. Enjoy with a simple roasted chicken, with Indonesian Chicken Saté (see page 244), or as part of a vegetarian meal, coupled with basmati rice and lentils.

Stir-Fried Broccoli and Shiitake Mushrooms

Results of a large study conducted by the National Cancer Institute suggested that eating more fruit and vegetables, such as broccoli, reduces the risk of cancer of the mouth and throat, types of cancer associated with heavy drinking. Shiitake mushrooms also fight cancer.

YIELD: 4 SERVINGS

$^1/_4$ cup dried shiitake mushrooms
2 tablespoons unrefined safflower oil
1 (2-inch) piece fresh ginger, peeled
  and minced

1 clove garlic
$1^1/_2$ pounds broccoli florets
Salt

1. Soak the mushrooms in 1 cup of hot water. When tender, drain, reserving the liquid. Trim the mushrooms and cut into bite-size pieces.

2. Set a wok or large skillet over medium-high heat and heat for 2 to 3 minutes. When hot, add the oil, ginger, and garlic. Stir-fry for 30 seconds.

3. Add the broccoli and mushrooms. Raise the heat to high and stir-fry the vegetables for 5 minutes, until the broccoli turns bright green and begins to brown.

4. Season with salt and a couple of tablespoons of the mushroom-soaking liquid. Continue to stir-fry until almost all liquid has evaporated and the broccoli is tender. Serve immediately.

Italian-Style Spinach
(Menu 11)

This gutsy mix of flavors, based on a classic Italian recipe, makes eating your greens a welcome assignment. Also try substituting kale for the spinach, another healing leafy green full of minerals, but cook the kale longer, at least 15 minutes.

YIELD: 4 SERVINGS

2 pounds fresh spinach
3 tablespoons golden raisins
1 clove garlic

3 tablespoons extra-virgin olive oil
2 anchovies

1. If using bunched spinach, cut off the root end. Fill the kitchen sink with several inches of water and submerge the spinach. Swish around, letting any soil that may be clinging to the leaves drop to the bottom. Repeat with fresh water until the leaves are clean. Or use bagged, prewashed and cut spinach, and simply give a quick rinse. Remove and discard any dark, soggy leaves or discolored stems.

2. In a small bowl, soak the raisins in warm water for 10 minutes to soften and plump. Chop the garlic separately.

3. Fill a medium-size pot with water, bring to a boil, and add the spinach. Cook for 3 minutes, drain thoroughly, and set aside.

4. In a large skillet, heat the oil and add the garlic, raisins, and anchovies. Sauté over medium heat for 5 minutes. Add the spinach and season with salt and pepper.

5. Cover and cook for 5 to 10 minutes to combine the flavors. Serve hot or at room temperature as an antipasto.

Pan-Fried Tomatoes
(Menu 10)

These quick-cooking fresh tomatoes, with their succulent texture, are sure to become a breakfast favorite, served with eggs, or English-style with beans on toast.

YIELD: 4 SERVINGS

4 medium-size tomatoes
1 cup bread crumbs, preferably whole wheat

$1/2$ teaspoon thyme
3 tablespoons extra-virgin olive oil
Salt and pepper

1. Core the tomatoes and cut crosswise in $1/2$-inch slices.

2. Scatter the bread crumbs on a large plate, and sprinkle the thyme over them. Season with salt and pepper.

3. Put the olive oil in a skillet over medium-high heat. Dredge each tomato slice in bread crumbs, coating both sides, and place in the hot oil.

4. As the slices of tomato begin to brown, turn with a spatula and fry the other side, for a total cooking time of no more than 10 minutes. Serve immediately.

Sautéed Kale
(Menu 13)

Kale is one of the dark leafy greens, along with collards and beet greens, which are high in calcium. A variation on this recipe is to make it with a combination of these greens.

YIELD: 6 SERVINGS
2 pounds kale
1 yellow onion
4 cloves garlic
$1/4$ cup extra-virgin olive oil
Kalamata olives (optional)
Lemon juice (optional)

1. Wash, trim, and chop the kale. Chop the onion and slice the garlic.

2. Put the oil in a heavy-bottomed skillet and add the onion. Cook over medium heat for 5 minutes. Stir in the garlic and cook for 1 minute. Add the kale.

3. Cover the skillet and cook for 15 minutes, or until the kale begins to wilt. Season with salt and pepper. And the addition of some pitted kalamata olives and a squeeze or two of lemon juice won't hurt! Also consider replacing the kale with broccoli rabe, a gourmet vegetable that's a favorite in Italy.

Sautéed Sweet Red Peppers
(Menu 14)

In traditional Chinese medicine, red peppers are considered a "fire" food, stimulating energy. Have a serving and see if you can sense their get-up-and-go energy.

YIELD: 4 SERVINGS
4 red bell peppers
2 tablespoons extra-virgin olive oil
Salt and pepper
2 tablespoons balsamic vinegar

1. Stem and seed the peppers and cut into strips.

2. Heat the oil in a large skillet set over medium-high heat for about a minute and add the peppers. Cook, stirring occasionally, until the peppers are very tender and lightly browned, 15 to 20 minutes. Season with salt and pepper.

3. Add the vinegar and stir the peppers. Cook over low heat for an additional 2 minutes. Enjoy with goat cheese spread on whole-grain crackers. Try the brand of crackers called Ak-Mak.

Greek-Style Green Beans
(Menu 18)

Sample the flavors in this vegetable dish and you'll be asking for seconds. Remember, one of the nutrition goals for recovery is to eat more vegetables.

YIELD: 4 SERVINGS
1 pound green beans, stem ends
    trimmed
1 (15-ounce) can tomatoes
$1/4$ teaspoon ground cinnamon
Salt and pepper

1. Set a collapsible steamer over an inch or two of water in a large pot. Cut the green beans into $1^1/2$-inch lengths and put in the steamer.

2. Cover; cook the beans for about 5 minutes, until somewhat tender.

3. Transfer two-thirds of the green beans to a skillet. Reserve and refrigerate the remaining green beans for Tuna Salade Niçoise (see Note). Add the tomatoes and cinnamon, and stir to combine. Simmer for 30 minutes, uncovered, adding liquid if necessary. Season with salt and pepper.

Note: This recipe calls for enough green beans to generate leftovers. You can save cooking time and have some of these beans for lunch the next day, using them in the recipe for Tuna Salade Niçoise (see page 223). Reserve one-third of the beans you've just cooked.

Oven–Baked "Fries"
(Menu 15)

There's no need to deep-fry when oven-baked potato sticks can taste as good as these. You'll also spare yourself the trans fats in fried oil.

YIELD: 4 SERVINGS
2 russet potatoes
2 sweet potatoes
1 egg
2 tablespoons extra-virgin olive oil, plus
    extra for oiling the baking sheet
Salt and pepper

Preheat the oven to 450°F.

1. Scrub the potatoes but don't peel them. Slice the potatoes lengthwise into $1/2$-inch slabs and then cut into sticks.

2. Whisk together the egg and olive oil in a medium-size bowl. Add the potatoes and toss to coat on all sides.

3. Oil a baking sheet and arrange the potatoes, separating each stick. Bake, turning occasionally, until golden and crunchy, about 35 minutes. Season with salt and pepper.

Boiled Potatoes ✷
(Menu 18)

If you want some regular white potatoes, have new potatoes with their crisp, waxy texture. They have less of an effect on blood sugar than do russets, which have a higher starch content.

YIELD: 4 SERVINGS
$1^1/2$ pounds new potatoes, skins on
    and scrubbed (see Note)
Dash of olive oil
Parsley, minced, for garnish

1. Bring a pot of salted water to a boil. Lower the heat to medium so the water boils gently; add the potatoes and cook until tender, about 40 minutes, depending on size.

2. Drain the potatoes and return two-thirds of them to the pot. (Reserve and refrigerate the remaining potatoes for Tuna Salade Niçoise [see Note].) Add the olive oil. Cook the potatoes over very low heat, occasionally shaking the pan, about 5 minutes, until there is no visible moisture.

3. Dust the potatoes with minced parsley and serve.

Note: The amount of potatoes called for in this recipe is enough for four at dinner, plus extra that you can use to make Tuna Salade Niçoise, page 223 the next day. Reserve about one-third of the potatoes.

Baked Sweet Potatoes 𝒲
(Menu 7)

For blood sugar control, sweet potatoes are a better choice than white potatoes because they have less of an effect on blood glucose.

YIELD: 4 SERVINGS
4 medium-size sweet potatoes
3 tablespoons butter substitute, such
   as Smart Balance Buttery Spread
Ground cinnamon or ginger (optional)

Preheat the oven to 450°F.

1. Line a baking pan with aluminum foil to catch the syrupy juice that the potatoes release as they cook.

2. Place the potatoes in the pan and, using a fork or knife, pierce each potato a few times to keep the skins from bursting. Bake for about 1 hour, along with the turkey breast recommended for this menu (see page 247 for recipe), until the potatoes are very tender and soft.

3. Serve with butter substitute and a pinch of ground cinnamon or ginger.

Soups

The Recipes:

Egg Drop Soup ⓦ
Nearly Instant Curried "Squash" Soup ⓦ
"Cream" of Asparagus Soup ⓦ
Mexican Gazpacho Soup
Salad Bar Minestrone Soup ⓦ
Lentil Soup with Prosciutto ⓦ
Cream of Cauliflower Soup with Rosemary and Thyme
Thai Coconut-Chicken Soup
Shiitake Mushroom Soup ⓦ

Soups are ideal foods for recovery, full of nourishing vegetables, simmered poultry and meats, whole grains, and legumes. As the ingredients cook and release their nutrients, these end up in the broth. Thankfully, there's no such thing as a deep-fried soup, and homemade versions don't need to be loaded with salt like the commercial kinds. Just stay away from creamed soups, with their saturated fat, to support your liver as it mends. If you're in the first days and weeks of abstinence, having soup for lunch or dinner can be a particularly good choice. During this period, you may have trouble digesting foods and even not much of an appetite. A warming bowl of soup could feel just right.

Egg Drop Soup 🍲
(Menu 4)

This easy-to-make soup gives you fortifying protein. Start with a bowlful when you're having Salad Bar Stir-Fry (see page 240) as a main course.

YIELD: 2 SERVINGS
1 egg
3 cups chicken broth

1. Whisk the egg in a small bowl and set aside.

2. In a saucepan, heat the broth, bringing it almost to a boil. Lower the heat to medium.

3. Slowly pour the whisked egg into the broth. Briefly stir with a fork and let the soup cook for 1 more minute. When the soup is done, the streamers of egg in the broth will be cooked through and fully set. Serve immediately.

Nearly Instant
Curried "Squash" Soup 🍲
(Menu 13)

This tastes like squash soup but you start with canned pumpkin, a time and effort saver. Like squash, pumpkin is also loaded with vitamin A and the spices in curry are anti-inflammatory.

YIELD: 4 SERVINGS
1 (28-ounce) can pumpkin puree
(not pumpkin pie filling)
1 (28-ounce) can low-sodium
chicken broth

1 tablespoon curry powder,
preferably sweet Madras style
1 tablespoon butter

1. Put the pumpkin puree, chicken broth, curry powder, and butter in a medium-size pot. Bring nearly to a boil, lower the heat to medium, and cook for 15 minutes to combine the flavors. Serve with a peanut butter and banana sandwich for a great flavor combo.

"Cream" of Asparagus Soup 🍲
(Menu 5)

Asparagus is a recovery vegetable because it's a source of B vitamins and vitamin C as well as calcium and magnesium, all possibly deficient for a person in recovery.

YIELD: 4 SERVINGS
1 pound asparagus
1 onion
1/4 cup rolled oats or mashed potato
4 cups low-sodium chicken or
    vegetable broth

1. Trim the asparagus and peel and dice the onion. Put the asparagus, onion, oats, and broth in a medium-size pot. Bring to a boil, lower the heat, and cook, covered, for 15 minutes.

2. In batches, puree the cooked vegetables and broth in a blender or food processor, transferring each blenderful to a bowl.

3. Return the puree to the pot and season with salt and pepper. Cook for an additional 3 minutes to warm the soup and blend the flavors.

Mexican Gazpacho Soup
(Menu 11)

The clean, simple flavors of this soup are yours to enjoy without doing any cooking. Just chop and process to feed yourself quality ingredients, the mainstay of recovery eating.

YIELD: 4 SERVINGS

1 cucumber
2 pounds tomatoes
1/4 cup chopped red onion
Juice of 1 lime

3 tablespoons extra-virgin olive oil
1/2 teaspoon ground cumin
Salt
Tabasco sauce

1. Peel and coarsely chop the cucumber. Trim and quarter the tomatoes. Put the cucumber, tomato, onion, lime juice, olive oil, and cumin in a bowl and mix together.

2. Put a few cups of the mixture at a time in a food processor or blender and process until just slightly chunky. Transfer to a bowl and continue to process the remaining ingredients.

3. Season with salt and Tabasco sauce, and chill in refrigerator for at least 1 hour before serving.

Salad Bar Minestrone Soup ⚉
(Menu 15)

By collecting the vegetables and other ingredients for this soup from your supermarket's salad bar, you eliminate the prep work and only buy as much as you need. Have fun and invent your own combinations.

YIELD: 2 MEAL-SIZE PORTIONS

About $1/2$ cup each of 8 salad bar items, such as red beans, garbanzo beans, soybeans, cherry tomatoes, broccoli, cauliflower, beets, bell peppers, peas, spinach, mushrooms, onions, celery, and carrot

4 cups reduced-salt chicken or beef broth

2 tablespoons tomato paste

1 clove garlic

$1/2$ teaspoon dried oregano

2 ounces pasta (any shape)

Salt and pepper

Parmesan cheese

1. Put the salad bar ingredients, broth, tomato paste, garlic, and oregano in a large pot. Cook over medium heat for 15 minutes.

2. Add the pasta and cook for an additional 30 minutes, until the vegetables become soft. Season with salt and pepper. Serve topped with Parmesan cheese.

Lentil Soup with Prosciutto 🐟

Lentils are recommended by both the American Institute for Cancer Research and the American Heart Association. While canned lentil soup often tastes quite good, there's nothing like the fresh flavors of homemade. If you don't happen to have prosciutto, use regular ham instead. For the vegetarian version, use vegetable broth instead of chicken and skip the ham.

YIELD: 4 SERVINGS

1 cup brown lentils
5 cups low-fat chicken broth
1 (15-ounce) can diced tomatoes with juice
3 ounces prosciutto, diced
$1/2$ cup finely chopped onion
4 cloves garlic, peeled and minced

$1/2$ teaspoon ground cumin
$1/8$ teaspoon dried oregano
2 tablespoons extra-virgin olive oil
1 tablespoon lemon juice
$1/4$ teaspoon Tabasco sauce
Salt and pepper

1. Wash the lentils and spread them out on a white plate to pick over for bits of stone and other debris.

2. Put the lentils, chicken broth, tomatoes, prosciutto, onion, garlic, cumin, and oregano into a large pot. Bring the mixture to a boil over high heat, uncovered, stirring occasionally. Lower the heat to low and cook until the lentils are tender but not mushy, 45 minutes to 1 hour.

3. In a small bowl, mix together the olive oil, lemon juice, and Tabasco. Stir into the soup and cook for an additional 5 minutes. Ladle into individual soup bowls and serve immediately.

Cream of Cauliflower Soup
with Rosemary and Thyme

This elegant soup fights cancer and dampens inflammation, thanks to the cauliflower and leeks. Enjoy it hot in the winter and chilled in the summer.

YIELD: 6 SERVINGS

2 leeks
1 head cauliflower
1 stalk celery
1 teaspoon dried rosemary

1 teaspoon dried thyme
2 cups 2% milk
1 tablespoon butter
Salt and pepper

1. To trim and wash the leeks, first remove the tough green leaves. Then cut off the root end, slice the leeks lengthwise in half, almost to the root end, and finally, spread out the leaves. Hold the leeks under running water and spread the cut layers, fanning them like a hand of cards. Now fill a large bowl with water and slosh the root end of the leeks up and down to allow any remaining sand to drop to the bottom. Cut leeks into 4-inch-long sections.

2. Trim and chop the cauliflower and celery.

3. Put the leeks, cauliflower, and celery in a large pot. Add the rosemary, thyme, and 4 cups of water. Bring to a boil. Lower the heat to low, cover, and cook, stirring occasionally, for about 20 minutes.

4. Remove from the heat and puree the vegetables, using a food processor or blender. Puree in batches, transferring each batch to a bowl.

5. Return the soup to the pot. Add the milk and butter. Stir to combine. Season with salt and pepper. Serve.

Thai Coconut–Chicken Soup

This is the homemade version of a Thai restaurant standard offering, tom kha gai, *but in this case, by using light coconut milk, you control the amount of saturated fat, important for recovery.*

YIELD: 4 SERVINGS

1 russet potato	1 tablespoon chopped fresh cilantro
3 carrots	3 tablespoons extra-virgin olive oil
1 stalk celery	1 cup light coconut milk
3 boneless, skinless chicken breast halves	Salt
1/2 lemon	Red pepper flakes

1. Peel and dice the potato. Peel and slice the carrots. Trim and slice the celery. Cut the chicken into bite-size pieces. Put the chicken and 6 cups of water into a large pot and add the potato, carrots, and celery.

2. Zest the lemon and add to the pot, along with the lemon juice. Add the cilantro and olive oil.

(recipe continues, next page)

3. Bring the water to a boil over high heat and lower the heat to medium-low so that the water simmers. Cook the chicken and vegetables until tender, about 30 minutes.

4. Add the coconut milk and season with salt and red pepper flakes. Stir to combine and simmer an additional 3 minutes. Serve immediately.

Shiitake Mushroom Soup 🥄

Shiitake mushrooms contain a compound called lentinan, which fights virus infection and cancer.

YIELD: 6 SERVINGS

3 tablespoons unrefined safflower oil
1 cup diced yellow onion
1 cup chopped celery
2 tablespoons finely chopped fresh dill
2 cups (about 4 ounces) sliced shiitake mushrooms
2 cups (about 4 ounces) sliced button mushrooms
3 cups 2% milk
2 tablespoons whole wheat flour
Salt and pepper

1. In a large pot set over medium heat, put 2 tablespoons of oil, and the onion, celery, and dill. Cook until the vegetables have softened, stirring occasionally, about 10 minutes.

2. Add the shiitake and button mushrooms and sauté until tender, stirring occasionally, about 7 minutes. Add 2 cups of the milk and simmer the soup over low heat, uncovered.

3. Meanwhile, put 1 tablespoon of the oil in a small skillet and heat over medium heat. Add the flour, thoroughly mix with the oil, using a fork, and cook for 2 minutes, stirring frequently. Add the remaining 1 cup of milk and cook, stirring until smooth and thickened, about 3 minutes.

4. Add the milk mixture to the soup. Season with salt and pepper. Simmer for 10 minutes and serve.

Salads

The Recipes:

Greek Salad
Orange and Walnut Salad
Carrot Slaw
Danish Apple-Beet Salad
Grilled Salmon on Toasted Corn and Lima Bean Salad
Chicken Salad with Avocado and Papaya
Tuna Salade Niçoise
Celery Root in Mustard-Tarragon Dressing
Ratatouille
Fancy Shrimp Salad

These salads are made with a variety of recovery ingredients including beets, carrots, lima beans, avocado, oranges, chicken, and tuna. Such dishes are an especially easy way to add vegetables to your meals and eaten raw offer more vitamins and minerals than their cooked versions. Salads are also low-tech dishes, requiring only simple kitchen skills like chopping, slicing, and tossing. Even if you're only just beginning to do some of your own cooking, you can make a salad!

Greek Salad
(Menu 1)

Because of the feta cheese, which gives you some protein and fat, this salad makes a satisfying meal. If you think you aren't a salad eater, try this two-fisted combination of flavors.

YIELD: 4 SERVINGS

1 large tomato
1 scallion
4 heaping cups romaine lettuce (bagged, precut lettuce or head of romaine)
8 stuffed grape leaves, canned or fresh from the deli
12 olives, preferably kalamata olives

$1/2$ pound feta cheese (feta is sold in blocks or bagged and already crumbled; sample the stronger Greek-style feta and the milder French-style feta.)
Greek bottled salad dressing or homemade (page 268), or oil and vinegar

1. Cut the tomato into eight wedges and cut the scallions crosswise into small bits.

2. On each lunch plate, place 1 cup of chopped lettuce. Arrange the tomato slices, grape leaves and olives on lettuce. Crumble one-fourth of the cheese over each salad and sprinkle with chopped scallion.

3. Drizzle with salad dressing. If using just oil and vinegar, add a couple of pinches of dried oregano, and the dressing will taste Greek!

Orange and Walnut Salad
(Menu 1)

The walnuts supply you with omega-3 fats, which keep the brain and heart healthy, while the oranges, with their membranes and pith, provide bioflavonoids. These help balance hormone levels that, according to research, drinking beer or bourbon can affect. These two alcoholic beverages contain phytoestrogens that alter hormone status.

YIELD: 4 SERVINGS

1 small head Boston lettuce
2 oranges
$1/3$ cup chopped walnuts

Bottled vinaigrette dressing or homemade Walnut Oil Dressing (page 272)

1. Wash and trim lettuce, tear leaves into bite-size pieces.

2. Peel, seed, and cut oranges into chunks.

3. Put the lettuce, oranges, and walnuts into a bowl and toss. Drizzle with dressing, toss again, and serve.

Carrot Slaw
(Menu 3)

This salad gives you plenty of roughage to improve poor digestion, sometimes an issue in recovery.

YIELD: 6 SERVINGS
3 cups shredded carrot
1^1/$_2$ cups chopped celery
^{1}/$_4$ cup raisins
^{1}/$_2$ cup mayonnaise

1. Put the carrot, celery, and raisins in a bowl and toss to combine.

2. Add the mayonnaise and toss to coat the other ingredients. Serve slightly chilled.

Danish Apple–Beet Salad
(Menu 8)

Beets are a recovery vegetable because they contain betaine, a compound that may help prevent fatty infiltration of the liver.

YIELD: 4 SERVINGS

1 Golden Delicious apple
1 (15-ounce) can whole beets
^{1}/$_4$ cup mayonnaise

2 tablespoons prepared mustard
1 tablespoon honey
^{1}/$_2$ teaspoon dried dill

1. Core and cut the apple into small chunks.

2. Drain the beets and cut into bite-size pieces.

3. In a medium-size bowl, mix together the mayonnaise, mustard, honey, and dill.

4. Add the apple and beets, and toss to combine the ingredients. Serve chilled.

Grilled Salmon on Toasted Corn and Lima Bean Salad
(Menu 12)

Any salad can be topped with fresh-off-the-grill meat or fish to create a substantial meal. Try this recipe for salmon salad and Steak Salad, page 253.

YIELD: 4 SERVINGS

12 cherry tomatoes
1 scallion
3 tablespoons extra-virgin olive oil
2 ears corn (2 cups)
1 cup frozen lima beans, defrosted
$1/2$ teaspoon fresh summer savory
Salt and pepper
4 (4-ounce) portions of salmon fillets
　(see Note)
1 lemon

1. Halve the tomatoes and finely chop the scallion.

2. Put the olive oil in a large skillet set over medium-high heat. Add the corn and scallion and cook until the corn just begins to brown and smells faintly like popcorn, about 5 minutes.

3. Lower the heat to medium and add the tomatoes, lima beans, and summer savory. Cook until the ingredients are heated through and the flavors begin to blend. Season with salt and pepper. Set aside and keep warm.

4. Meanwhile, heat a lightly oiled skillet or ridged pan. Put the salmon fillets into the pan and cook for 3 to 4 minutes on each side, until the salmon is cooked through. Remove from the heat and keep warm.

5. To assemble the salad, spoon a portion of the corn mixture onto each dinner plate and top with the grilled salmon. Squeeze lemon juice over the fillets. Serve immediately.

Note: Wild salmon is far preferable to farmed salmon, which contains higher levels of toxins and heavy metals, and is given feed that contains pharmaceuticals. Spare your liver the chore of detoxifying these.

Chicken Salad with Avocado and Papaya
(Menu 17)

Start with a store-bought chicken salad and slice up some avocado and papaya, to turn yourself into a gourmet cook—a great confidence builder for timid cooks to do more healthy home-cooking and not just order in pizza.

YIELD: 4 SERVINGS

1 avocado
1 papaya
1 pound ready-made chicken salad
8–12 leaves of Boston lettuce

1. Peel the avocado, remove the pit, and cut lengthwise into $1/2$-inch-wide slices. Peel the papaya, scoop out the seeds, and cut lengthwise into 1-inch-wide slices.

2. To serve the salads, lay two or three lettuce leaves on each plate. Place a scoop of chicken salad in the center. Arrange the avocado and papaya around the chicken salad and serve.

Tuna Salade Niçoise
(Menu 19)

You can make this salad from scratch, first cooking the potatoes and green beans, or have these two vegetable for dinner the night before, and then the next day turn them into this classic French Mediterranean salad. See pages 209 and 210 for guidance on how to generate these useful leftovers.

YIELD: 4 SERVINGS

$1/2$ pound cooked new potatoes
$1/3$ pound cooked green beans
2 tablespoons capers
3 (6-ounce) cans chunk light tuna
  packed in water

$1/4$ cup extra-virgin olive oil
1 tablespoon balsamic vinegar
1 teaspoon prepared mustard
$1/2$ teaspoon dried basil, or 2 sprigs
  fresh, leaves only

(recipe continues, next page)

1. Slice the potatoes and cut the green beans into 1-inch lengths. Put the potatoes, beans, and capers into a large bowl. Drain the tuna and add to the vegetables, using a fork to break the fish into chunks.

2. In a small bowl, whisk together the oil, vinegar, mustard, and basil.

3. Drizzle the dressing over the tuna and vegetables. Gently toss to combine. Season with salt and pepper, and serve with a pesto baguette (see Note).

Note: If you want to take this salad to work, do what caterers do to save time on the day of an event and assemble sections the night before. Have the salad dressing ready and the potatoes, beans, and capers mixed in a bowl. Then in the morning, add the tuna and the dressing to the vegetables and toss.

Celery Root in Mustard–Tarragon Dressing

Like celery, celery root, also known as celeriac, is a cleansing vegetable, acting as a diuretic. Although it may look to be very hard, celery root can be easily shredded in a food processor. Enjoy this classic of the French hors d'oeuvres tray and add variety to your diet.

YIELD: 4 SERVINGS
1 medium-size celery root
1/2 cup mayonnaise
2 tablespoons freshly squeezed
    lemon juice
1/2 teaspoon prepared mustard
1/4 teaspoon dried tarragon
Salt and pepper

1. Pare off the fibrous outside of the celery root. Cut the root into chunks and feed through the tube of a food processor fitted with the shredding blade.

2. In a medium-size bowl, mix together the mayonnaise, lemon juice, mustard, and tarragon. Add the celery root and toss to thoroughly coat. Season with salt and pepper. Chill and serve garnished with minced parsley.

Ratatouille

Now that this French dish is known worldwide, thanks to the movie of the same name, how about cooking some and savoring its earthy flavor? This vegetable stew is made with several recovery ingredients, including onions, garlic, tomatoes, and peppers. Enjoy it warm or at room temperature, as a main-course cooked "salad" for lunch, with bread and goat cheese on the side.

YIELD: 6 SERVINGS
1 medium-size onion
1 medium-size eggplant
1 orange bell pepper
1 red bell pepper
1 medium-size zucchini
4 tomatoes
2 cloves garlic
$1/4$ cup extra-virgin olive oil
Salt and pepper
3 sprigs fresh basil, leaves only,
   chopped (See Note)

1. Peel the onion, cut into $1/4$-inch slices, and cut these in half; peel the eggplant, slice horizontally, and cut in bite-size pieces; core, seed, and dice the peppers; trim the zucchini and cut horizontally in $1/2$-inch slices; trim, seed, and coarsely chop the tomatoes; crush the garlic, remove its skin, and mince.

2. Put the olive oil and onion into a large pot with a tight-fitting lid. Cook over medium-low heat, stirring occasionally, until the onion begins to soften and become translucent, about 7 minutes. Add the garlic and cook for 2 minutes.

3. Add the eggplant, peppers, zucchini, tomatoes, and $1/2$ cup of water. Season with salt and pepper and stir gently to combine. Over medium heat, cook, covered, stirring occasionally, until the vegetables have softened, about 1 hour. Add the fresh basil and cook for an additional 15 minutes. Season with additional salt and pepper, if necessary.

Note: If using dried basil, add 1 teaspoon along with the vegetables in Step 3.

Fancy Shrimp Salad

You'll think you ordered this salad from the menu at a fine hotel, when you taste this shrimp cloaked in the elegant dressing. This dish also offers recovery benefits. Shrimp is a source of selenium, a trace mineral that aids detox and enhances the antioxidant effects of vitamin E.

YIELD: 4 SERVINGS
$1/4$ cup celery, chopped finely
1 scallion, sliced thinly
1 clove garlic, minced
1 tablespoon chile sauce
$1/2$ teaspoon dry mustard
$1/4$ cup tarragon vinegar
$1/4$ cup unrefined safflower oil
$1^1/2$ pounds defrosted frozen jumbo
    shrimp, cooked, shelled, and
    deveined
Juice of 1 lemon
1 teaspoon paprika
Salt and pepper
1 (10-ounce) bag mixed gourmet
    salad greens, or about 2 cups
    loosely packed greens per serving

1. Put the celery, scallion, garlic, chile sauce, mustard, and vinegar into a jar with tightly fitting lid.

2. Stir the oil into the vinegar mixture, a little at a time. Close the jar and shake vigorously until the dressing is thoroughly blended. Refrigerate for 2 to 3 hours to chill.

3. Slice the defrosted shrimp, halving them lengthwise. Put the shrimp into a bowl. Sprinkle with lemon juice and paprika. Season with salt and pepper.

4. To assemble the shrimp salad, place 2 cups of lettuce on each plate. Divide the shrimp among the servings. Pour the chilled dressing over the shrimp and serve. Garnish with slices of apple or cucumber, preferably English cucumber, for a clean, fresh taste.

Fish and Shellfish

The Recipes:

Tuna Fish Cakes with Spicy Mustard Mayonnaise
Garlic Shrimp
Tilapia Tacos
Crispy Cod Fillets 🕸
Baked Halibut with Prosciutto and Herbs 🕸
Mediterranean Fish Stew
Grilled Red Snapper with Anchovy and Caper Sauce
Salmon Fillets with Ravigote Sauce
Grilled Halibut with Tapenade
Scallop Seviche with Avocado

In terms of good nutrition for recovery, fish deserves to be the featured food of a meal, be it breakfast, lunch, or dinner, at least twice a week. Seafood is rich in minerals, a more reliable source than foods grown on the land if that land has been overfarmed and depleted of minerals. Finfish such as halibut, flounder, bass, and cod are sources of calcium, iron, magnesium, potassium, and selenium, as well as zinc. Seafood is also a source of all the B vitamins and two fat-soluble vitamins, A and D, especially abundant in fatty fish such as tuna and salmon.

Oilier fish are also the top sources of two special omega-3 fatty acids, EPA (eicosapentaenoic acid) and DHA (decosahexaenoic acid). These oils are especially beneficial for recovery and, at the same time, the recovering alcoholic is likely to be deficient in them. Researchers who measured DHA in the brains of individuals with a history of drinking found its levels to be reduced by 50 percent from what is considered normal.

You may already be familiar with EPA and DHA if you're in the habit of taking nutritional supplements. These fish oils are widely sold in capsule form as more and more of their health benefits are being discovered. EPA and DHA thin the blood, preventing blood clots from forming, and reduce inflammation. They are found in abundance in the adrenal glands, sex glands, and eyes. And there is a very high level of DHA in the nervous system and brain, where DHA plays an important role in communication between cells. Emerging evidence indicates that alcohol may initiate inflammation of neurons in the brain, leading to brain damage, another reason for increasing your intake of these oils for their anti-inflammatory effect.

Avoiding Toxins in Fish

For the same reasons that going organic makes sense for recovery, you want to eat fish with the lowest levels of both pesticides and toxic metals, such as cadmium and mercury, which damage the kidneys and nervous system and can lead to cancer. Good rules to follow are:

▶ Consume a variety of fish.
▶ Eat fish with an offshore habitat, such as flounder, sole, ocean perch, haddock, halibut, and cod.
▶ Favor smaller fish. These fish, which are younger, haven't had the time to accumulate a lot of toxins compared with their older counterparts.

According to the federal Food and Drug Administration and the Environmental Protection Agency, the following big fish contain higher levels of mercury:

▶ Shark
▶ Swordfish
▶ King mackerel
▶ Tilefish

In addition albacore tuna, which is white, has more mercury than does canned chunk light tuna, which comes from smaller fish.

Making Sure Fish Is Fresh

Seafood requires special attention when it comes to freshness. Fresh fish has a better flavor and texture than fish that is not, since it dries out quickly. Fish also has a short shelf life and can spoil in a day or two, especially if mishandled. Follow these tips on shopping for seafood and keeping it fresh once you've brought it home.

Whether you're considering purchasing a whole fish displayed on a bed of ice at a fancy fish store, or you're about to buy a tidy little fillet wrapped up in plastic at your usual supermarket, you need to know what fresh fish looks like.

Signs that a whole fish is fresh:

▸ Skin glistens.
▸ Scales are intact.
▸ Gills are red or pink, not gray, brown, or green.
▸ Eyes are firm and convex, not sunken.
▸ Flesh is somewhat resistant when gently pressed.

Signs that a fillet is fresh:

▸ Flesh is luminous and translucent.
▸ Fillet is firm and elastic to the touch.

Plan to do your fish shopping as your last errand, then go directly home and immediately put it away in your refrigerator for that night's dinner. Or if you need to cook it the next day, be sure the seafood is kept at 39°F or lower. You can also store fish on a bed of ice, using a suitable container that allows drainage of the melting ice water. A small metal roasting pan that has some holes perforated in it, placed in a larger pan, would suffice.

The seafood that gives you the most fish oils per serving are the following:

▸ Salmon

▸ Tuna

▸ Mackerel

▸ Sardines

▸ Herring

▸ Anchovies

▸ Caviar

The recipes in this section give you the chance to see how good fish can be.

Tuna Fish Cakes with Spicy Mustard Mayonnaise

Be sure to buy chunk light tuna, which contains lower amounts of mercury than does white albacore. Chunk light also has richer flavor that can stand up to the spicy mustard sauce recommended with this dish.

YIELD: 4 SERVINGS

$^1/_4$ cup unrefined safflower oil, plus extra if needed for cooking fish cakes
$^1/_4$ cup finely chopped onion
2 tablespoons capers
1 tablespoon chopped fresh parsley

1 cup cooked mashed potatoes
3 (6-ounce) cans chunk light tuna
3 tablespoons whole wheat flour
1 egg, slightly beaten
$^1/_2$ cup seasoned whole-grain bread crumbs

1. Heat 1 tablespoon of the oil in a small skillet and add the onion. Cook over medium heat for about 5 minutes, until the onion becomes translucent.

2. Transfer the onions to a large bowl. Add the capers and parsley, and stir. Add the potato and tuna, and gently mix.

3. Shape the tuna mixture into eight cakes. Distribute the flour on a work surface or large plate; beat the egg in a wide, shallow bowl; spread out the bread crumbs on another surface or large plate. To seal the cakes and create an appetizing crust, dip each tuna cake in the flour, next in the egg, and lastly in the bread crumbs.

4. Heat the remaining 3 tablespoons of oil in a skillet. When hot, add several tuna cakes, about four at a time, to not crowd the pan. Cook over medium-high heat for about 4 minutes each side, until the crust is crunchy and golden. Cook the cakes in batches, adding more oil if necessary. Place the cooked cakes on paper towels to drain off the excess oil. Serve with Spicy Mustard Mayonnaise (see page 263).

Garlic Shrimp
(Menu 9)

Instead of deep-fried shrimp and all the batter and oil that comes with it, relax with a bowlful of shrimp sautéed with a pungent combination of parsley, garlic, and red pepper flakes, ingredients that all have healing properties.

YIELD: 4 SERVINGS

1/2 bunch fresh parsley or cilantro, leaves only, to yield 1/2 cup pureed
4 cloves garlic, peeled
2 tablespoons extra-virgin olive oil

1/2 teaspoon red pepper flakes, or to taste
1 pound large shrimp, peeled and deveined

1. Put the parsley and garlic in a food processor and puree.

2. Heat the oil in a skillet over medium heat and add the pepper flakes; toast them for a few seconds.

3. Add the shrimp and stir-fry for 2 minutes. Add the garlic mixture, lower the heat, and continue to cook, stirring frequently, until the shrimp are opaque, 3 or 4 minutes. Serve immediately.

Tilapia Tacos

One of the easiest ways to sell a fish dinner to someone who is timid about seafood is to tuck some fish into a crunchy, spiced-up taco. This one comes with a good portion of recovery vegetables.

YIELD: 4 SERVINGS

2 tablespoons extra-virgin olive oil, plus extra for coating the skillet
1 medium-size onion, peeled and sliced thinly
1–2 chile peppers, such as serrano or jalapeño, chopped finely
1/2 teaspoon dried oregano, preferably Mexican
1/2 teaspoon ground cumin
1 large sweet pepper (red, yellow, or orange), cut into thin strips
2 sprigs fresh cilantro, leaves only, minced
1 clove garlic, minced
Salt and pepper
1 pound tilapia fillets
8 corn tortillas
1 cup shredded cabbage

1. Warm 2 tablespoons of the oil in a skillet set over medium-high heat. Add the onion, chile pepper, oregano, and cumin, and cook for 3 minutes, stirring frequently.

2. Add the sweet pepper and cilantro. Cook the mixture for 10 minutes, until it begins to soften, then add the garlic. Cook for an additional 1 to 2 minutes, stirring occasionally, until the garlic cooks but does not brown. Season with salt and pepper. Set aside and keep warm.

3. Meanwhile, as the vegetables are cooking, oil a skillet or grill pan and set over medium-high heat. Add the fish. Cook for 3 to 5 minutes per side, depending on the fillets' thickness. When done, cut into small chunks. Set aside and keep warm.

4. To heat the tortillas, set batches of four on a plate, sprinkling a few drops of water on each before laying down the next, and microwave for 1 minute per batch. Heat a serving platter.

5. To assemble the tacos, lay a tortilla flat and place about 1/4 cup (2 ounces) of tilapia in the center of the tortilla. Sprinkle some shredded cabbage over the fish and then spoon 1/4 cup of the sautéed vegetables over this. Fold the filled tortilla in half and transfer to a heated platter. Continue to fill and fold the remaining tortillas.

6. Serve two tortillas per portion along with such condiments as avocado slices, salsa, and wedges of lime.

Timing Fish

Here is a general rule to follow in preparing fish to make sure you've cooked it enough, but not so much that it dries out: cook fish for 10 minutes per inch of thickness measured at the fish's thickest point.

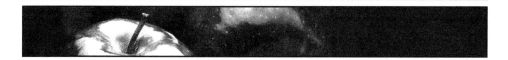

Crispy Cod Fillets 🐟
(Menu 15)

Like the tuna cakes recipe, this recipe employs a useful technique for breading any variety of fish or other foods. The cod is coated first with the flour, next with eggs, and then with bread crumbs, creating a double barrier around the fish and lots of crunch.

YIELD: 4 SERVINGS

$^1/_2$ cup all-purpose flour
2 eggs
$^1/_2$ cup plain bread crumbs
$1^1/_2$ pounds cod (2 fillets, or 1 large
   fillet cut into pieces)

Salt and pepper
2 tablespoons unrefined safflower oil

1. Spread the flour on a large plate. Beat the eggs in a wide, shallow bowl. Spread the bread crumbs on another large plate.

2. Heat a large skillet over medium-high heat for 2 to 3 minutes.

3. Meanwhile, season the cod fillets with salt and pepper. Dredge the cod in the flour, shaking off any excess, and then dip in the eggs. Finally, dip the cod fillets in the bread crumbs.

4. Pour the oil into the skillet. Lowering the heat to medium, cook until the fillets are browned on both sides, turning once. Cook for a total of 10 to 15 minutes. When the fish is done cooking, it will have lost its translucency but should still be firm and juicy.

5. Serve immediately, with Oven-Baked "Fries" (see page 210), ready-made deli coleslaw, bottled tartar sauce, and wedges of lemon.

Baked Halibut with Prosciutto and Herbs 🐚

A way of braising foods in French cooking is to set the fish or meat on a bed of chopped vegetables, called a mirepoix in French. This recipe makes use of this technique but increases the amount of vegetables, to give you more nutrients and fiber and make a complete meal. For this recipe you can use any one of a variety of mild-flavored, thick white fish, including cod, halibut, and orange roughy.

YIELD: 4 SERVINGS

3 tablespoons extra-virgin olive oil
3 cloves garlic, minced
1 bulb fennel, trimmed and cut into thin slices
2 carrots, peeled and sliced crosswise into rounds
2 parsnips, peeled and sliced crosswise into rounds
1 medium-size onion, peeled and cut into thin slices
4 waxy potatoes, peeled and cut into $1/2$-inch dice
4 slices prosciutto, cut into strips
$1/4$ teaspoon dried oregano

$1/4$ teaspoon dried rosemary
$1^1/2$ pounds halibut fillet
Salt and pepper
2 cups unsalted chicken or vegetable broth, or water

Preheat the oven to 375°F.

1. On the bottom of a casserole, drizzle 1 tablespoon of the oil and then sprinkle the minced garlic over the oil.

2. Add about half of the fennel, carrots, parsnips, onion, potatoes, prosciutto, oregano, rosemary, and halibut. Season with salt and pepper.

3. Drizzle another tablespoon of the oil over the fish and then add the remaining vegetables, prosciutto, herbs, and fish. Again season with salt and pepper. Pour the broth over the vegetables and fish, and add the remaining oil.

4. Cover the casserole and bake for about 45 minutes, until the potatoes and fish are cooked through. Serve in shallow pasta bowls along with some of the broth.

Mediterranean Fish Stew
(Menu 20)

Cooking fish in a seasoned broth, as in this recipe, guarantees success every time, the liquid keeping the fish moist and adding flavor.

YIELD: 4 SERVINGS

$^1/_2$ pound spicy turkey sausage
$^1/_2$ medium-size onion
1 clove garlic
$^1/_2$ pound spinach
2 tablespoons extra-virgin olive oil
1 (15-ounce) can tomatoes
4 (4-ounce) pieces of fish such as cod or
   halibut, or a mix of these (see Note)
3 cups chicken broth
1 cup orzo, or other pasta shape of
   your choice

1. Remove the sausage skin and cut the sausage into $^1/_2$-inch chunks. Peel and chop the onion and garlic. Trim, wash, and chop the spinach.

2. Heat the oil in a large stockpot and add the sausage and onion. Cook over medium heat for 3 to 4 minutes.

3. Add the garlic, tomatoes, fish, chicken broth, and pasta. Cook for 10 to 15 minutes, or until the fish is cooked through.

4. Transfer the fish to a platter and cover with aluminum foil to keep warm.

5. Stir the spinach leaves into the sauce, raise the heat to medium-high, cover the pot, and cook for 2 minutes. Remove the pot from the heat. To serve, place the fish in individual serving bowls and spoon the stew over the fish. Serve immediately with a fresh green salad.

Note: While this stew requires a meaty fish, which holds up best in liquid, more delicate fish, such as red snapper and shrimp, can also be included. Add these toward the end of the cooking process, as they need less time to cook; about 10 minutes for red snapper and 3 to 4 minutes for shrimp.

Grilled Red Snapper with Anchovy and Caper Sauce

This recipe gives you a double serving of omega-3s, thanks to the red snapper and the anchovies.

YIELD: 6 SERVINGS

1 medium-size bunch flat-leaf parsley, leaves only, minced
1 (2-ounce) can anchovies, drained and minced
2 cloves garlic, peeled and minced
2 tablespoons capers, drained

Juice of 1 lemon
3/4 cup extra-virgin olive oil, plus extra for oiling the pan
Pepper
6 small red snapper
Arugula or baby spinach leaves

1. In a medium-size bowl, put the parsley, anchovies, garlic, capers, lemon juice, and olive oil. Using a fork, mix all ingredients together thoroughly. Season with pepper. Set aside.

2. Cook the fish on a preheated outdoor grill or a ridged grill pan on the stove top. Oil the cooking surface. Grill the fish according to their size and thickness. A reliable rule-of-thumb is to cook fish for 10 minutes for each inch of thickness. Small snapper should be done in 5 to 10 minutes.

3. To serve, arrange the greens on a large platter. Place a bowl of anchovy sauce in the center and arrange the individual fish around it. Serve each snapper with a portion of greens and a large spoonful of the sauce.

Salmon Fillets in Ravigote Sauce

Think salsa and translate that into something French and you have Ravigote sauce, based on a mixture of chopped raw tomatoes and onion. Serve this with that classic of healthful eating, poached salmon, for the anti-inflammatory effects of the oils in the fish, and for the anti-inflammatory compounds in the sauce's onions and garlic.

YIELD: 4 SERVINGS

1 ripe tomato, chopped finely
1/4 onion, peeled and chopped
2 scallions, trimmed and chopped
2 sprigs fresh parsley, leaves only, chopped
1 clove garlic, minced

1 tablespoon capers
1/4 cup extra-virgin olive oil
2 tablespoons fresh lemon juice
4 salmon fillets, 1/3 pound each
3/4 cup vegetable broth or water

1. Put the tomato, onion, scallions, parsley, garlic, capers, olive oil, and lemon juice in a bowl. Stir to combine and set aside.

2. Arrange the fillets, skin side down, in a skillet and add the broth. Over medium-low heat, simmer, covered, until the salmon is done, 8 to 10 minutes per inch of thickness. Test for doneness by inserting a thin-bladed knife into the fish to check that the salmon flesh has turned opaque.

3. Transfer the steaks to individual dinner plates. Use a paper towel to sponge up any liquid that collects around the fillets. Spoon the sauce over the salmon and serve immediately.

Grilled Halibut with Tapenade
(Menu 18)

This quick recipe pairs a savory jarred condiment with fish, a gourmet touch that requires little effort. Use this sauce with other meaty fish like halibut, to preserve the balance of complementary flavors.

YIELD: 4 SERVINGS

2 tablespoons prepared tapenade
2 tablespoons extra-virgin olive oil
1¹/₂ pounds halibut
2 tablespoons unrefined safflower oil

Special equipment: Sixteen 6-inch wooden skewers

1. Place the skewers in a container and fill with water until the skewers are completely covered. Soak the skewers for 30 minutes to prevent them from burning as the fish cooks.

2. In a small bowl, combine the tapenade with the olive oil and set aside.

3. Rinse the halibut and dry with paper towels. Slice the fish into bite-size chunks and skewer about three pieces per kabob. Then, to prevent the fish from slipping and turning, thread each kabob with a second skewer parallel to the first. To ensure even cooking, make sure that chunks of fish are separated along the skewers.

4. Heat a ridged grill pan or a large skillet over medium heat and coat cooking surface with the safflower oil, raising the heat to medium-high. Add the fish

(recipe continues, next page)

and cook on one side until golden brown, 5 to 6 minutes, occasionally shaking the pan to keep the fish from sticking.

5. Turn the kabobs, using cooking tongs. Cook the fish on second side for 4 to 5 minutes. Serve immediately, garnished with the tapenade sauce.

Scallop Seviche with Avocado

For this warm-climate dish, the scallops are "cooked" not by heat but by the acids in the lime juice. Like other shellfish, scallops contain only a scant amount of saturated fat but deliver a variety of minerals.

YIELD: 4 SERVINGS AS A MAIN COURSE

8 limes or more, to yield at least 1^1/$_2$
    cups lime juice
^{1}/$_2$ cup finely chopped red onion
2 cloves garlic, minced
1 pound bay scallops (the smaller
    kind of scallops)
^{1}/$_2$ pound cherry tomatoes, halved
1 avocado, peeled, pitted, and diced
1 tablespoon chopped fresh cilantro
2 tablespoons extra-virgin olive oil
Salt and pepper

1. Squeeze the limes, collecting the juice in a bowl. Pour the juice through a strainer set over a shallow baking dish to remove seeds and collect the juice in the container. Add the onion and garlic to the baking dish and stir to combine.

2. Add the scallops to the baking dish, making sure the fish is spread out in as even a layer as possible and that there is enough lime juice to cover the scallops. Squeeze more lime juice if necessary.

3. Loosely cover the scallops and refrigerate for a minimum of 5 hours, or until the scallops become opaque. Stir the scallop mixture occasionally to make sure the fish "cooks" evenly.

4. Drain the scallops. Add the tomatoes, avocado, cilantro, and olive oil. Toss gently to combine. Season with salt and pepper. Enjoy a serving for lunch, along with steamed corn tortillas, and as a first course at dinner or a party hors d'oeuvre with scallops and cherry tomato halves threaded on bamboo skewers.

Poultry

The Recipes:

Salad Bar Stir-Fry
Oven-Fried Chicken 🐚
Slow-Cooked Tarragon Chicken
South American–Style Chicken with Corn Pudding
Chicken with Tons of Garlic
Indonesian Chicken Saté
Chicken Curry
Chinese Chicken Salad
Baked Turkey Breast 🐚
Turkey Tonnato

Like seafood, chicken and turkey are mainstays of recovery eating when it comes to animal sources of protein. A prime virtue of poultry is that, compared with red meat, it's relatively low in fat, since fatty liver is made worse by a high-fat diet. It's also lower in saturated fat, which also increases the risk of infiltration of liver tissue. While almost half of the fat in beef can be saturated, saturated fat makes up only about one-third of the fat in white meat chicken. Furthermore, most of the poultry fat is in the skin, which you can easily remove before or after cooking.

Chicken and turkey are also excellent sources of B vitamins, which deserve special attention for recovery. Alcohol impairs the absorption and use of many B vitamins and increases their excretion. Both chicken and turkey are especially high in vitamin B_6 and niacin, which have special benefits for the heart. Poultry also supplies selenium, a trace mineral essential in the detox chemistry that takes place in the liver. A $3^1/2$-ounce portion of dark meat turkey supplies almost 60 percent of the recommended daily allowance (RDA).

The following ten recipes give you a wide variety of ways to prepare these birds, from quick stir-fry to long simmered dishes. There's a healthy version of fast-food fried chicken and sophisticated Turkey Tonnato. Start

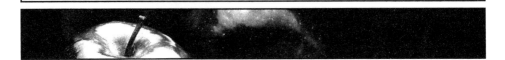

with one of these entrées and add some of the many vegetable, grain, and bean side dishes in this chapter, and you can invent many a tasty meal.

Salad Bar Stir-Fry
(Menu 4)

You'll never look at a salad bar the same way again. It's not just raw food; it's ingredients for cooking!

YIELD: 1 SERVING

$2/3$ pound salad bar ingredients, including pieces of cooked chicken and vegetables such as broccoli florets, slices of green pepper, sliced mushrooms, cucumber slices, chopped celery, and chopped scallion

2 tablespoons hoisin sauce
2 tablespoons unrefined safflower oil
1 tablespoon toasted sesame oil
2 tablespoons peanuts
1 tablespoon soy sauce

1. Put the chicken pieces in a bowl and toss with 1 tablespoon of the hoisin sauce. Set aside.

2. Put 1 tablespoon of the safflower oil and the sesame oil in a skillet or wok. Heat the oil over high heat until the surface of the oil begins to shimmer. Add the vegetables. Stir-fry for about 4 minutes, using a spatula to quickly stir and toss the vegetables. Transfer the vegetables to a bowl.

3. Put the remaining tablespoon of safflower oil and the chicken in the skillet. Stir-fry for about 3 minutes, until the chicken is heated.

4. Return the vegetables to the pan. Add the peanuts, soy sauce, and the remaining tablespoon of hoisin sauce. Stir-fry for about 1 minute to reheat the vegetables and combine all the ingredients. Serve immediately. Enjoy with brown rice and Egg Drop Soup (see page 213).

Note: Also consider these stir-fry add-ins: pecans, shrimp, tofu, water chestnuts, shiitake mushrooms, bok choy, minced garlic, and grated ginger.

Oven-Fried Chicken 🐾

This is a handy cooking technique to know when you want fried chicken but not all the fat.

YIELD: 4 SERVINGS

1 cup whole wheat bread crumbs
$1/4$ cup unrefined safflower oil
2 eggs
1 tablespoon prepared mustard
1 teaspoon dried thyme
1 teaspoon salt

$1/2$ teaspoon pepper
1 chicken, cut into parts, skin removed

Preheat the oven to 400°F.

1. Take a sheet pan or a baking sheet and line it with aluminum foil for easy cleanup later. Set a large, flat wire baking rack on the pan or sheet.

2. Put the bread crumbs in a shallow dish. Drizzle the oil over the crumbs. Using a fork, mix thoroughly.

3. In a second bowl, combine the eggs, mustard, thyme, salt, and pepper.

4. Dip a piece of chicken in the egg mixture and turn on both sides to coat. Then place in the bread crumbs. Sprinkle the crumbs over the top, pressing on them so they adhere to the chicken. Turn the piece of chicken over and do the same on the other side. Place on the baking rack. Repeat with the other pieces of chicken.

5. Bake for 40 minutes, or until the outside of the chicken browns and its juices run clear. Pile in a basket lined with paper napkins and you can pretend you're having take-out, but a healthier, homemade version.

Slow-Cooked Tarragon Chicken

The process of detoxifying alcohol uses up the body's supply of zinc. Chicken is a good source of zinc and also supplies niacin, another nutrient that may be deficient because of drinking too much.

YIELD: 4 SERVINGS

1 carrot, sliced
1 stalk celery, sliced
1 turnip, peeled and cut into wedges
1 fennel bulb, sliced
$1/2$ teaspoon dried tarragon
$1/2$ cup whole wheat flour, for
   dredging chicken
1 teaspoon salt
$1/4$ teaspoon pepper
2–3 pounds chicken parts, including
   thighs, most of the skin removed

1 tablespoon extra-virgin olive oil
$3/4$ cup water or chicken broth
Special equipment: slow-cooker or
   Crock Pot

1. Put the carrot, celery, turnip, fennel, and tarragon in the bottom of a slow-cooker or stoneware insert of a Crock Pot and mix together.

2. On a large plate, combine the whole wheat flour, salt, and pepper. Dredge the chicken pieces in the seasoned flour.

3. Heat the olive oil in a large skillet. Over medium-high heat, brown the chicken.

4. Place the chicken on top of the vegetables. Add the water. Cover and cook for about 6 hours on low. The chicken is done when its juices run clear when pierced. Spoon the chicken and vegetables into a large serving dish and serve.

South American–Style Chicken with Corn Pudding

This casserole, with origins in the traditional cuisine of Bolivia, is testimony to the intriguing flavors and wholesome ingredients commonly found in time-honored dishes. The combination of chicken and eggs provides plenty of protein to help rebuild body tissues in recovery.

YIELD: 6 SERVINGS

1 chicken, about 3 pounds, cut into pieces
2 tablespoons extra-virgin olive oil
1 onion, peeled and chopped finely
1 (15-ounce) can tomatoes
12 small green olives, stuffed with pimiento
1/3 cup raisins
1/4 teaspoon ground cinnamon
Salt and pepper
The topping:
4 cups corn kernels, fresh or frozen
4 tablespoons butter substitute, such as Smart Balance Buttery Spread
2 teaspoons sugar
4 eggs
Paprika

1. Put the chicken in a large pot and fill with water to just cover the chicken. Bring the water to a boil. Lower the heat to medium and cook, partially covered, for 45 minutes, or until the chicken is tender. Let the chicken cool in the chicken stock. (To easily remove most of the saturated fat in the stock, refrigerate the pot of chicken overnight; the next day, spoon the hardened fat from the surface of the stock.) Remove and discard the skin and bones and cut the chicken into bite-size pieces.

2. In a large skillet, heat the olive oil and add the onion. Cook, stirring occasionally, until the onion softens, about 5 minutes.

3. Add the tomatoes to the onion and cook for 5 minutes. Add the olives, raisins, cinnamon, and chicken. Season with salt and pepper. Set aside.

Preheat the oven to 350°F.

4. To make the topping, puree the corn in a food processor. In a saucepan, melt the butter substitute. Add the corn puree and sugar, and stir to combine. Season with salt. Beat in the eggs, one at a time. Over very low heat, cook the topping, stirring constantly with a wooden spoon, until the corn mixture begins to thicken. Remove from the heat.

5. To assemble the dish, spoon about one-third of the corn mixture into a casserole dish. Add the chicken mixture and then the remaining topping. Sprinkle with paprika.

6. Bake the chicken casserole for 1 hour, until the topping is lightly browned and set. This dish tastes even better the next day and it's also a great make-ahead choice for entertaining.

Chicken with Tons of Garlic

This dish lets you savor garlic in quantity, like a side serving of vegetables. Garlic, which is known to have an anti-inflammatory effect, is more potent raw than cooked, but certainly eating nearly a dozen cloves in a serving can still do you some good. Give slow-cooked whole garlic a try and you'll be surprised by its aromatic, mild flavor.

YIELD: 4 SERVINGS

1 chicken, cut into parts, drumstick and thigh separated
2 tablespoons extra-virgin olive oil
2 stems fresh parsley, leaves only, chopped finely
2 bay leaves
1 teaspoon dried rosemary
$1/2$ teaspoon dried thyme
Salt and pepper
At least 2 heads of garlic, or about 40 cloves

1. Put the chicken, olive oil, parsley, bay leaves, rosemary, and thyme in a casserole or large saucepan. Season with salt and pepper. Open the heads of garlic and separate the cloves, keeping the skins intact. Add to the chicken mixture. Add $1/2$ cup of water and mix together.

2. Set over medium-high heat and bring to a boil. Cover with a tight-fitting lid and lower the heat to low.

3. Cook for about 1 hour, until the garlic and chicken are very tender.

4. Transfer to a serving bowl and garnish with parsley. Serve this dish with crusty multigrain bread. Squeeze the cloves of garlic out of their casings and spread it on the bread like butter. Enjoy.

Indonesian Chicken Saté
(Menu 10)

Recovery eating includes appealing party foods like chicken saté. Serve it with sweet and tart Asian Cucumber Salad (see page 264).

YIELD: 4 MAIN COURSE SERVINGS, 6 IF SERVED AS AN APPETIZER

1 (2-inch) length fresh ginger
1 cup light coconut milk
2 tablespoons fresh lime juice
2 teaspoons curry powder
$1^{1}/2$ pounds chicken breast tenders
$3/4$ cup prepared peanut sauce
Special equipment: about twelve bamboo skewers, 12-inch for barbecue grill or 6-inch for ridged grill pan

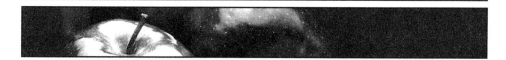

1. Peel the ginger and chop finely. Put the ginger, coconut milk, lime juice, and curry powder in a small bowl and stir to combine into a marinade.

2. Put the chicken in a sealable plastic bag, add the marinade, and turn the bag to coat the chicken. Squeeze the bag to eliminate the air and seal. Refrigerate for 1 to 3 hours to allow the chicken to marinate.

3. Meanwhile, soak the bamboo skewers in water for 30 minutes to prevent the wood from burning while cooking the chicken.

4. Thread each chicken tender on a skewer and place on a preheated outdoor grill or on a ridged grill pan on the stove top. Cook the chicken until lightly browned, about 5 minutes, then turn and cook for an additional 5 minutes. Serve with prepared Asian peanut sauce.

Chicken Curry
(Menu 21)

This one-pot dish gives you a substantial meal with little effort and tastes even better on the next day or two. Make enough for leftovers, one way to make sure you'll eat three meals a day, Goal 1 of this nutrition recovery program.

YIELD: 4 SERVINGS

4 large chicken breast halves
1 medium-size onion
2 medium-size potatoes
2 tablespoons crystallized ginger

1 (15-ounce) jar Indian curry sauce
1/4 cup pecans
1 tablespoon Madras curry powder
   (optional)

(recipe continues, next page)

1. Cut the chicken into bite-size chunks. Peel and dice the onion. Peel and quarter the potatoes. Chop the ginger into small bits.

2. Pour the curry sauce into a large pot. Add an equal amount of water and stir. Put the chicken, onions, potatoes, ginger, pecans, and optional curry powder in the pot.

3. Cook over medium heat, partially covered, stirring occasionally, for 1 hour, or until the chicken and potatoes are cooked through and the flavors blend. Add more water if necessary. Serve as is or with brown basmati rice and Indian side dishes such as lentils and pureed spinach, which are sold already prepared, packaged in aluminum packets, and only require quick reheating.

Chinese Chicken Salad

Certain foods like iceberg lettuce and cucumbers are mostly water and may taste especially good to you if you're newly abstinent. Alcohol is dehydrating, as anyone knows who has suffered a hangover. This salad, served in restaurants, is usually coated with a supersweet dressing and topped with deep-fried noodles, giving you an extra dose of fat. Here's a healthier version you can toss together at home.

YIELD: 4 SERVINGS

4 chicken breast halves, skin removed
1/2 cup unrefined safflower oil
1/4 cup toasted sesame oil
1/4 cup soy sauce
1/4 cup seasoned rice vinegar
1 (1-inch-long) piece fresh ginger,
   peeled and minced
1 head iceberg lettuce
4 scallions
1/2 cucumber, preferable English
   cucumber
1 (8-ounce) can sliced water chestnuts

2 cups beansprouts
1/4 cup peanuts

1. Put the chicken breasts into a medium-size saucepan and cover with water. Bring to a boil and lower the heat to medium. Poach the chicken until tender and cooked through, 20 to 25 minutes. Let the chicken rest in the broth until cool enough to handle. Cut into bite-size pieces.

2. Meanwhile make the dressing by whisking together in a bowl the safflower oil, sesame oil, soy sauce, rice vinegar, and ginger. Set aside.

3. To prep the vegetables: shred the iceberg lettuce; trim and cut the scallions crosswise into $1/4$-inch slices; peel the cucumber, remove and discard the seeds, and cut into bite-size pieces.

4. Put the chicken, lettuce, scallions, cucumber, water chestnuts, and beansprouts in a bowl. Toss to combine. Add the dressing and toss again.

5. Distribute the salad on dinner plates. Garnish with the peanuts and serve.

Baked Turkey Breast 🦃
(Menu 7)

Be sure to collect the cooking juices when you bake this turkey and serve the bird au jus. B vitamins are water soluble and make their way out of the meat in these juices.

YIELD: 6 SERVINGS, PLUS LEFTOVERS
1 (3-pound) turkey breast, skin
   removed
3 tablespoons extra-virgin olive oil
$1/2$ teaspoon dried rosemary
Salt and pepper
1 teaspoon butter

Preheat the oven to 450°F.

1. Coat the turkey breast with the olive oil. Season with the rosemary, salt, and pepper. Wrap in aluminum foil and place the turkey breast in a roasting pan.

2. Put the turkey in the oven and roast for 1 hour and 15 minutes, or until an instant-read thermometer indicates that the turkey meat has reached a temperature of 160°F. To brown the turkey, a few minutes before it is done, partially open the foil wrap and spread the butter on top surface of the turkey breast.

3. Let rest 10 minutes before slicing. Serve with Baked Sweet Potatoes (see page 211) and a mix of peas and pearl onions. This vegetable combo is sold frozen in most supermarkets.

Turkey Tonnato Salad

A novel way of preparing turkey is to serve it with tuna sauce, a variation on a classic Italian dish, Vitello Tonnato, made with veal. Cloaked under the sauce, white meat turkey successfully masquerades as veal and is a less expensive and more humanely raised alternative. This dish is served at room temperature, an ideal lunch or light supper especially in warm weather.

YIELD: 4 SERVINGS

1 pound sliced breast of turkey (home-baked, not deli-style sliced turkey)
$^1/_2$ cup mayonnaise
1 (6.5-ounce) can chunk light tuna, packed in water, drained
3 anchovies

1 tablespoon capers, drained
1 tablespoon lemon juice
Pepper
4 cups washed arugula leaves or other lettuce
Lemon wedges, for garnish

1. Put the turkey slices in a pot with enough water to cover. Poach over medium heat, about 15 minutes, until the meat juices run clear when pierced. Allow to cool in the cooking liquid.

2. To make the sauce, put the mayonnaise, tuna, anchovies, capers, and lemon juice in a food processor fitted with a metal blade. Process until blended but not completely smooth. Season with pepper.

3. Distribute the lettuce among dinner plates. Arrange the turkey slices on the lettuce. Spoon about 3 tablespoons of tuna sauce over each serving of turkey. Garnish with lemon wedges.

Beef, Lamb, and Pork

The Recipes:

Pan-Fried Steak with Mustard Sauce
Turkish Meatballs
Beef Stroganoff
Steak Salad
Crock Pot Beef Stew
Barley-Lamb Soup
Moroccan Lamb
Pork Chops with Sautéed Onion and Apple

Protein is needed to repair the body in recovery and meat is an excellent source, supplying all the amino acids. Both chronic and acute misuse of alcohol causes reductions in protein synthesis in the heart, bone, skin, and small intestine. Ethanol also increases the excretion of nitrogen, the key component of protein, resulting in a loss of skeletal muscle protein. Up to two-thirds of alcoholics suffer this nitrogen loss. And when an alcoholic is also malnourished, lack of protein can quickly stop the liver from making albumin, a substance that affects fluid balance; accumulation of fluid results.

Foods like beef, pork, and lamb also provide the full range of B vitamins as well as zinc, nutrients that may be deficient in a person with a history of drinking. In addition, meat is a source of glutathione, a compound that helps convert fat-soluble toxins into water-soluble forms that the body can more readily excrete. This action gives support to a liver in recovery, strengthening its detox function. The liver also has the task of metabolizing amino acids. The following recipes provide moderate servings of protein to limit what the liver must handle.

Pan–Fried Steak with Mustard Sauce

Even if you don't regularly eat red meat, you may have one of those days when you're body tells you only a steak will do. Have a moderate-size portion and make sure to cook it right so it really satisfies your steak hunger. This recipe tells you how.

YIELD: 2 SERVINGS

1 boneless strip steak, or rib-eye steak, 1–1¼ inches thick, 8–10 ounces
Salt and pepper
1 tablespoon unrefined safflower oil
½ cup chicken broth

Pinch of dried rosemary
1 teaspoon prepared mustard
Special equipment: cast-iron skillet or stainless-steel skillet with an aluminum-core spatter screen (see Note).

1. Heat a skillet over medium heat for 10 minutes. Season the steak with salt and pepper.

2. When the skillet is heated, add the oil to the pan to coat the bottom. Place the steak in the pan and cover with a spatter screen. Cook the steak for 5 minutes on one side, until it is well browned, then turn it over to cook the other side. For a rare steak, cook for 3 more minutes; for medium-rare, 4 more minutes; and for medium, 5 more minutes.

3. Transfer the steak to a dinner plate and let rest for 5 minutes before serving.

4. Meanwhile, prepare the sauce. Using a paper towel, wipe the fat from the pan. Add the chicken broth. With a spatula, scrape the brown bits on the bottom of the pan, letting them dissolve in the broth. Add the rosemary and boil the broth until it reduces by half.

5. Add the mustard, stirring to combine. Spoon the sauce over the steak and serve immediately.

Note: You can certainly cook a steak without owning a spatter screen, a round mesh screen with a handle, which prevents hot fats from spattering all over your stove top, but you'll be glad you own one.

Turkish Meatballs
(Menu 17)

Here's a fresh take on hamburger, giving it Middle Eastern flavorings. Enjoy with generous helpings of the several vegetarian side dishes served with this dish, which are described in Menu 17 on page 146.

YIELD: 4 SERVINGS
1/4 cup plain bread crumbs,
    preferably whole wheat
1/4 cup milk
1 egg
1 tablespoon fresh mint leaves,
    chopped finely
1/4 teaspoon ground cinnamon
1/4 teaspoon ground allspice
1 pound ground beef
Salt and pepper
Oil for coating the roasting pan

Preheat the oven to 375°F.

1. Soak the bread crumbs in the milk for about 5 minutes, until the milk is absorbed. In a large bowl, lightly beat the egg. Add the mint leaves, cinnamon, allspice, and bread crumbs. Mix thoroughly with a fork. Add the beef and combine.

2. Divide the beef mixture into thirds and form four meatballs with each, for a total of twelve meatballs. Oil the bottom of a roasting pan and arrange the meatballs in the pan.

3. Bake the meatballs for about 25 minutes. Serve with Minted Yogurt (see page 146 in chapter 5).

Beef Stroganoff

There's room in recovery eating for guy food like this stroganoff, a beefy main course with lots of creamy sauce. You'd never know that almost half of it is mushrooms and the sour cream is nonfat.

YIELD: 4 SERVINGS

3 tablespoons butter substitute, such
    as Smart Balance Buttery Spread
1 tablespoon all-purpose flour
1 cup fat-free beef broth
1 pound beef tenderloin, trimmed,
    cut into thin slices and then into 1-
    inch pieces
Salt and pepper
$1/2$ cup finely chopped onion
$1/4$ teaspoon paprika
$3/4$ pound mushrooms, a mix of sliced
    button mushrooms and shiitake,
    cut into bite-size pieces
1 teaspoon dried dill
$1/4$ cup nonfat sour cream
1 teaspoon prepared mustard

1. In a skillet, melt $1^1/2$ tablespoons of the butter substitute over moderate heat. Add the flour and whisk constantly for 2 minutes. Add the broth in a slow stream, whisking constantly while bringing the broth to a boil. Lower the heat and simmer for 3 minutes, whisking occasionally. Set the sauce aside and cover to keep warm.

2. Season the beef with salt and pepper. Heat $1/2$ tablespoon butter substitute in a large skillet set over medium-high heat. Add the beef in two batches and cook until browned, about 1 minute for each batch. When done, the beef should still be pink inside. Transfer to a large bowl.

3. Put the remaining 1 tablespoon of butter substitute in the pan with the onions and paprika. Cook over medium heat, stirring occasionally, until the onions are golden, about 5 minutes. Add the mushrooms and cook, stirring occasionally, for 8 to 10 minutes, until the liquid they release has evaporated and the mushrooms have browned. Add the mushrooms to the cooked meat.

4. Put the sauce in the skillet. Whisk in the sour cream and mustard. Season with salt and pepper. Add the beef and mushrooms, and stir to combine. Serve over egg noodles.

Steak Salad
(Menu 16)

A modest portion of steak atop a salad can seem like more, mixed with lots of vegetables, but spares you the extra saturated fat that would come with a bigger portion.

YIELD: 2 SERVINGS

2 tablespoons extra-virgin olive oil
1 tablespoon balsamic vinegar
1 teaspoon soy sauce
1 clove garlic, minced
Salt and pepper

1 large tomato
2 heaping cups romaine lettuce
1/2 pound beef sirloin, about 1 1/2 inch thick
1/2 baguette

1. Make the salad dressing by whisking together in a small bowl the olive oil, vinegar, soy sauce, and garlic. Season with salt and pepper.

2. Slice the tomato and put in a large bowl along with the lettuce. Drizzle with the dressing and toss.

3. Broil or grill the steak. To broil, set the steak about 3 inches from the heat source and cook a total of 8 minutes for medium doneness. Place the steak on a cutting board and slice across the grain.

4. Arrange the salad on two dinner plates and top with the steak slices. Serve with a chewy multigrain baguette.

Crock Pot Beef Stew

Beef provides the full range of B vitamins, which are commonly deficient in alcoholics because drinking causes changes in the GI tract that lead to problems with absorption and use of these nutrients.

YIELD: 5 SERVINGS

1/4 cup whole wheat flour
Salt and pepper
1 1/4 pounds boneless beef stew meat, well trimmed of visible fat
2 tablespoons extra-virgin olive oil
2 carrots, peeled and cut into bite-size pieces
1 small onion, peeled and sliced

1 (15-ounce) can beef broth
2 tablespoons tomato paste
1 clove garlic, minced
1 bay leaf
1/2 teaspoon dried thyme
1/4 pound mushrooms, sliced
Special equipment: slow-cooker or Crock Pot

(recipe continues, next page)

1. Combine the whole wheat flour with the salt and pepper. Dredge chunks of beef in the seasoned flour.

2. Heat the olive oil in a large skillet and, over medium-high heat, brown the beef. Transfer to the Crock Pot, reserving the drippings in the skillet.

3. Put the carrot and onion in the skillet and brown, adding additional oil if necessary. Add to the Crock Pot.

4. Pour the beef broth into the skillet and deglaze the pan, using a spatula to scrape the brown bits from the bottom of the pan. Put into the Crock Pot along with the tomato paste, garlic, bay leaf, and thyme. Also stir in any remaining flour left from dredging the beef.

5. Cover and cook on low for 5 hours.

6. Adjust the seasoning and add the mushrooms. Continue to cook the stew for about 1 hour. Check for doneness of the meat, which should be fork tender. Serve with egg noodles.

Barley–Lamb Soup

This hearty cold-weather soup is a meal in itself. It's high in niacin, riboflavin, and vitamin B_{12}, thanks to the lamb, and the barley supplies soluble fiber, which stimulates the flow of bile, helping rid the body of toxins.

YIELD: 4 SERVINGS

1 (32-ounce) can fat-free, reduced-sodium beef broth, or similar boxed broth
1 cup pearled barley
1 pound lamb, from shoulder or leg, well trimmed of fat and cut into 1-inch cubes
1 medium-size onion
1 stalk celery, halved
3 carrots, sliced
2 teaspoons prepared mustard
$1/2$ teaspoon dried rosemary
Salt and pepper

1. In a large soup pot, combine the beef broth, barley, lamb, onion, and celery. Bring to a boil and lower the heat to low. Cook until the barley and lamb is tender, about 1 hour. Skim and discard any foam that rises to the top of the broth during cooking.

2. Discard the celery and add the carrots. Stir in the mustard and rosemary. Cook the soup for an additional 30 minutes. Season with salt and pepper.

3. Before serving, skim off any visible fat that may be floating on the surface of the soup. (You can also cool the soup and refrigerate overnight; then remove any white, hardened fat before reheating.) Correct the seasoning and serve.

Moroccan Lamb

Using a modern slow-cooker allows lamb to cook as if it were in a Moroccan tagine, a glazed earthenware casserole with a conical lid, used traditionally in Morocco to slowly cook meats. Prepared this way, the lamb is infused with an array of spices. A health note: lamb can be high in saturated fat, but this is no reason not to enjoy a moderate portion for dinner if you limit saturated fat at breakfast and lunch.

YIELD: 6 SERVINGS

1 1/2 pounds boneless lamb, preferably leg or shoulder
Salt and pepper
2 tablespoons extra-virgin olive oil
1 onion, chopped coarsely
2 cloves garlic, peeled and chopped finely
5 whole green cardamom pods
1 bay leaf
1 teaspoon ground cumin
1/2 teaspoon ground cinnamon
1/2 teaspoon ground ginger

1/2 teaspoon ground turmeric
1/2 teaspoon dried thyme
1/4 cup chopped fresh parsley
Pinch of cayenne
1 (14.5-ounce) can tomatoes
3 tablespoons tomato paste
1 (15-ounce) can chickpeas, drained and rinsed
Special equipment: slow-cooker or Crock Pot, and cheesecloth (see Note)

1. Trim away most of the visible fat off the lamb. Cut the meat into 1- to 1 1/2-inch chunks. Season with salt and pepper. Heat the oil in a large skillet over medium heat. Add the lamb and brown on all sides, working in batches if necessary. Transfer to a bowl.

2. Add the onion to the skillet and cook, stirring occasionally, until the onion softens, about 5 minutes. In the last minute of cooking, add the garlic. Put the onion and garlic in the slow cooker.

3. Add the cardamom pods and bay leaf, tied into a small square of cheesecloth. Add the cumin, cinnamon, ginger, turmeric, thyme, parsley, cayenne, tomatoes, tomato paste, chickpeas, and 1/2 cup of water. Cover and cook on low for 5 hours, or until the lamb is fork tender. Remove the cardamom seeds and bay leaf. *(recipe continues, next page)*

4. Serve the lamb with whole-grain couscous.

Note: Using cheesecloth to hold the seasonings is optional, but spares you the risk of biting down on a pungent cardamom pod or a bay leaf.

Pork Chops with Sautéed Onion and Apple
(Menu 14)

Loin chops, trimmed of fat, give you a relatively lean way to enjoy pork. Just remember to remove the visible fat.

YIELD: 4 SERVINGS

4 bone-in center loin pork chops, at least 1 inch thick
2 tablespoons extra-virgin olive oil
1 cup chicken broth, plus up to $1/2$ cup extra for sauce
1 tablespoon lemon juice
$1/2$ teaspoon dried rosemary
1 tablespoon prepared mustard
1 onion, thinly sliced
1 apple, cored and sliced

1. Trim away the excess fat from the chops and season with salt and pepper.

2. Heat a large skillet over medium-high heat for 2 to 3 minutes. Add 2 tablespoons of the olive oil and, when very hot, add the chops, raising the heat to high. Quickly brown the chops on both sides, about 3 minutes.

3. Lower the heat to medium and add $1/2$ cup of the broth, and the lemon juice and rosemary. Cook, turning the chops once or twice, until the liquid is all but evaporated. Add the remaining $1/2$ cup of broth.

Preheat the oven to 200°F.

4. Lower the heat to low and cover. Cook the chops until tender but not dry, 10 to 15 minutes. Transfer the chops to a platter and put in a warm oven.

5. Stir the mustard into the juices in the skillet and add the onion. Stir, cover, and cook over medium heat for 5 minutes.

6. Remove the cover and add the apple plus up to $1/2$ cup more broth, if there is not sufficient liquid to prevent burning. Cook until the onions soften and begin to turn golden and the apples soften, about 5 minutes. Pour over the chops and serve.

Sandwiches

The Recipes:

Grilled Cheese Sandwich ℳ
Meat Loaf Sandwich
Southwest Chicken Burger
Savory Salmon Sandwich
Turkey and Avocado Sandwich ℳ

Each of the following five sandwiches has a place in the recovery menus featured in chapter 5. If you don't feel like cooking a complete meal, you can still make one of these and know that you've taken a good step in nourishing yourself. These recipes are fairly basic—you can use them as starting points to come up with your own healthy sandwich combinations.

Grilled Cheese Sandwich 🍲
(Menu 4)

Enjoy this sandwich with onion soup (see page 118).

YIELD: 1 SERVING

2 slices whole-grain bread

3 ounces thinly sliced cheddar cheese

2 teaspoons unrefined safflower oil

1. Assemble the bread and cheese to make a sandwich.

2. Heat the oil in a small skillet. Put the sandwich in the skillet and weigh down with a heavy pot cover. Cook for 2 to 3 minutes over medium-low heat, until the bottom of bread is lightly browned.

3. Flip the sandwich and repeat, checking that the cheese has melted. Serve immediately with the onion soup.

Meat Loaf Sandwich
(Menu 12)

Start with ready-made meat loaf and make yourself a substantial lunch. Heat it up with vegetables such as sweet peppers, tomatoes, and onions to make this satisfying sandwich.

YIELD: 4 SERVINGS

1 green bell pepper, trimmed and seeded

1 onion, peeled

2 tablespoons extra-virgin olive oil

1 pound meat loaf

4 lunch rolls

1. Chop pepper and onion into bite-size pieces.

2. Heat the olive oil in a skillet, add the onion and pepper, and cook over medium heat, stirring occasionally, until the vegetables are quite soft, about 10 minutes.

3. Using your fingers, crumble the meat loaf into the skillet. Mix with the vegetables and heat through.

4. Split a sandwich roll, removing some of the inside bread, and fill the roll with the meatloaf combo. Chow down.

Southwest Chicken Burger
(Menu 11)

Look for chicken patties with a Southwest taste, such as Trader Joe's Chile Lime Chicken Burgers, for mouthwatering flavor.

YIELD: 1 SERVING

1 chicken patty	Lettuce leaves
2 slices whole-grain bread	Chile sauce

1. Preheat a lightly oiled skillet over medium-high heat. Place the chicken burger in the pan and cook for 3 to 4 minutes per side if the patty is defrosted (5 to 6 minutes per side if frozen), or according to the package instructions if a longer time is required.

2. Lightly toast the bread.

3. Spread the chile sauce on one of the slices of toast, top with the chicken and some lettuce, and close the sandwich with the other bread slice. Enjoy with Mexican Gazpacho Soup (see page 214).

Savory Salmon Sandwich
(Menu 5)

The appetizing flavors of this sandwich are a perfect match with "Cream" of Asparagus Soup (see page 214). This recipe makes a hefty amount of salmon salad for a hearty sandwich. If you have leftovers after making your sandwich, refrigerate and enjoy as a snack.

YIELD: 1 SERVING

1 (7.5-ounce) can salmon	Pinch of pepper
1 tablespoon chopped scallion	2 slices whole-grain bread
2 teaspoons balsamic vinegar	Leaf of Boston lettuce

1. Remove any unwanted skin and bones from the salmon.

2. Put the salmon, scallions, and vinegar in a bowl and mix with a fork. Season with pepper.

3. Spread the salmon mixture on one of the slices of bread, add the lettuce leaf, and close with the other bread slice.

Turkey and Avocado Sandwich 🍂
(Menu 8)

Turkey breast is low in fat and avocado is full of healthy ones, the mononounsaturated kind that are good for the heart. Avocados also deliver folic acid, a nutrient that may need replenishing in recovery.

YIELD: 1 SERVING
2 slices whole-grain bread
1 tablespoon cranberry sauce
1 tablespoon mayonnaise
4 ounces sliced turkey breast
3 slices peeled avocado
Salt and pepper

1. Spread one slice of bread with the cranberry sauce and the other with the mayonnaise.

2. On the bread slice with the cranberry, arrange the turkey and top with the avocado. Season with salt and pepper.

3. Close the sandwich with the second slice of bread. Cut in half and serve.

Condiments and Savory Side Dishes

The Recipes:

Fresh Tomato Salsa
Homemade Tortilla Chips
Spicy Mustard Mayonnaise
Garlic-Onion Dip
Asian Cucumber Salad
Moroccan Carrots Scented with Lemon and Spices
Sautéed Bananas
Yogurt Cheese 🔊
Spiced and Toasted Nuts

Recovery eating doesn't need stop with the main course. Condiments and savory little side dishes can also do you some good. Many of the ingredients that give them their flavor are also healing foods, such as garlic, onions, chiles, ginger, and mint. The following recipes show you how to make favorites like salsa and chips from scratch so you control the ingredients and also let you explore exotic dishes such as the Morocco-inspired spiced carrots.

Fresh Tomato Salsa
(Menu 2)

Each ingredient in salsa does its part in recovering health by easing digestion, enhancing immunity, and protecting against cancer. Salsa is a truly healing condiment.

YIELD: 1¹/₂ CUPS

1 tomato
¹/₄ medium-size onion
2 sprigs fresh cilantro or parsley,
   leaves only

1 small chile pepper such as serrano,
   or Tabasco sauce

1. Chop the tomato and onion into small bits. Finely chop the cilantro. Combine these in a small bowl.

2. Seed and mince the pepper and add, to taste, or season the tomato mixture with Tabasco sauce. Refrigerate, covered with plastic wrap, until ready to use.

Homemade Tortilla Chips
(Menu 2)

Make your own chips for dipping and spare yourself the refined oils in commercial brands. For extra flavor, sprinkle with chile powder.

YIELD: 8 SERVINGS

8 corn tortillas
Unrefined safflower oil, for oiling
   tortillas
Chile powder (optional)

Preheat the oven to 400°F.

1. Stack the tortillas and cut into eight wedges as you would a pie. Use an oil sprayer filled with unrefined safflower oil to lightly spray each side of the tortilla pieces. Sprinkle with chile powder, if desired.

2. Arrange in a single layer on an ungreased baking sheet and bake for 10 to 12 minutes, until golden.

Spicy Mustard Mayonnaise

Make sure to use mayonnaise that doesn't list partially hydrogenated fats on its label, to avoid trans fats. Serve with the Tuna Fish Cakes (see page 230).

YIELD: ABOUT 1 CUP
1 cup mayonnaise
1 tablespoon prepared mustard
2 teaspoons fresh lemon juice
Hot sauce

1. Combine the mayonnaise, mustard, and lemon juice in a small bowl.

2. Mix together thoroughly with a fork. Season to taste with the hot sauce.

Garlic-Onion Dip

This dip, which is based on yogurt, gives you a healing food for the digestive tract and lots of flavor. Keep on hand along with sliced raw veggies, for a refreshing, crunchy nibble.

YIELD: ABOUT 3 CUPS
3 cups plain yogurt
2 cloves garlic, peeled and minced
2 tablespoons minced onion
1 teaspoon lemon juice
2 teaspoons mustard powder
Salt and pepper

1. Put the yogurt in a bowl. Add the garlic, onion, lemon juice, and mustard powder. Stir to combine.

2. Season with salt and pepper. Store, covered with plastic wrap, in the refrigerator, so it will be ready for snacking.

Asian Cucumber Salad
(Menu 10)

Drinking leaves the body dehydrated. Especially in the early stages of abstinence, juicy foods are called for, such as the cucumber in this refreshing salad. It's the perfect condiment to have with Chicken Saté (see page 244).

YIELD: 2 CUPS
1 cucumber
$1/4$ red onion
1 tablespoon minced cilantro
$1/4$ cup seasoned rice vinegar
Salt and pepper

1. Peel the cucumber and cut crosswise into thin slices. Cut the onion into thin slivers.

2. Put the cucumber, onion, cilantro, and vinegar in a bowl. Mix well. Season with salt and pepper.

Moroccan Carrots Scented with Lemon and Spices

You won't need to be coaxed to eat your vegetables when you taste these scrumptious exotic carrots.

YIELD: 4 SERVINGS

5 medium-size carrots
3 cloves garlic
$1/4$ cup lemon juice
2 tablespoons extra-virgin olive oil
$1/2$ teaspoon ground cumin

$1/4$ teaspoon fennel seeds
2 sprigs fresh parsley
2 sprigs fresh cilantro
Salt and pepper

1. Peel the carrots. Cut in half crosswise and then quarter lengthwise. Crush the garlic cloves.

2. Bring water to a boil in a pot and add the carrots and garlic. Cook over medium-high heat until tender, about 20 minutes.

3. Meanwhile, put the lemon juice, olive oil, cumin, fennel seeds, parsley, and cilantro in a shallow bowl. Beat the ingredients with a fork to combine. Set the dressing aside.

4. Thoroughly drain the cooked carrots. Add to the dressing in the bowl. Gently mix to coat the carrots with the dressing. Season with salt and pepper, and mix once again. Enjoy immediately or, for the best flavor, refrigerate, covered, and serve later in the day at room temperature.

Sautéed Bananas
(Menu 9)

The bananas are sautéed in a small amount of butter for flavor. The butter also produces quick browning, eliminating the need for long cooking that would make the bananas too soft.

YIELD: 4 SERVINGS

2 firm bananas, or ripe (yellow-black) plantains if available

1 clove garlic
2 teaspoons butter

1. Peel the bananas. Cut in half lengthwise and in half again. Then cut in half crosswise. Mince the garlic.

2. Heat the butter in a skillet and add the bananas and garlic. Cook over medium heat, turning once with a spatula, until golden, about 10 minutes.

Yogurt Cheese 🔄
(Menu 21)

This recipe requires preparation the day before it's needed, as the yogurt is strained overnight. Use yogurt cheese as a dip for fresh vegetables. It's also the garnish for the frittata in Menu 21 (see page 153).

YIELD: 2 CUPS

2 cups low-fat plain yogurt
2 sprigs fresh mint, leaves only
2 teaspoons extra-virgin olive oil

Special equipment: piece of cheesecloth about 12 by 24 inches

(recipe continues, next page)

1. Dampen the cheesecloth. Fold in half to form a square and line a medium-size sieve with the cloth.

2. Pour the yogurt into the center of the sieve and set over a deep bowl or cooking pot. Loosely cover and refrigerate overnight to drain the liquid from the yogurt. Discard the liquid.

3. Spoon the thickened yogurt into a bowl. Add the mint and stir to incorporate. Garnish with the olive oil and serve.

Spiced and Toasted Nuts

Nuts are packed with vitamins and minerals and make a highly nutritious snack. Consider a moderate-size palmful a serving (12 to 14 nuts).

YIELD: 4 CUPS
1^1/$_2$ cups almonds
1 cup walnuts
1 cup cashews
2 tablespoons organic butter
2 teaspoons chile powder
^{1}/$_4$ teaspoon ground cinnamon
^{1}/$_4$ teaspoon ground ginger
Salt and pepper

1. Put the almonds, walnuts, and cashews in a bowl and mix.

2. Melt the butter in a skillet. Add the chile powder, cinnamon, and ginger and, over medium heat, toast the spices for about 30 seconds, stirring occasionally.

3. Add the nuts to the skillet. Stir to coat with the spices. Cook over medium heat for 5 to 7 minutes, stirring continuously, until the nuts are fragrant and lightly browned. Season with salt and pepper.

4. Immediately transfer the toasted nuts to a large platter and distribute evenly to allow the nuts to cool and their moisture to escape. When cool, store in an airtight glass jar. Set the jar where you're sure to see it every day and remember to eat a few nuts when you want a snack.

Nutritious Dressings

The Recipes:

Basic Vinaigrette with Flaxseed Oil
Greek Salad Dressing
Avocado Dressing
Anchovy Vinaigrette
Sesame-Yogurt Dressing
Tomato Vinaigrette
Lemon Vinaigrette
Walnut Oil Dressing

When you're in the first stage of beginning to eat better, as you begin your new life of abstinence, it's understandable that you'll reach for a bottle of ready-made salad dressing to save time and effort—and that's okay if it means you'll be eating more leafy greens. But you can go one step better and make your own salad dressing from scratch, which has some notable health advantages because you control the ingredients.

Commercial dressings are very likely to be made with refined oils, especially those that contain omega-6 fatty acids, which are already overabundant in the American diet. (You can read about why this is important in chapter 4.) They often also contain sugars, including high-fructose corn syrup and sometimes stabilizers and preservatives. Instead, make your own, with all top-quality ingredients. The following recipes call for the healthiest oils—extra-virgin olive oil, avocado oil, walnut oil, and flaxseed oil.

Basic Vinaigrette with Flaxseed Oil

Making a salad dressing with flaxseed oil gives you an extra dose of omega-3s.

YIELD: ABOUT ²/₃ CUP DRESSING

6 tablespoons extra-virgin olive oil
2 tablespoons flaxseed oil
2 tablespoons lemon juice or
    balsamic vinegar
Salt and pepper

1 shallot, peeled and minced
¹/₄ teaspoon dried herbs, such as
    thyme or fines herbes
1 capsule vitamin E (optional) (see
    Note)

1. Put the olive oil, flaxseed oil, and lemon juice into a small bowl. Beat with a fork to thoroughly combine.

2. Season with salt and pepper. Add the minced shallot and herbs, and mix again. Store the dressing in a sealed container in the refrigerator and use within the week.

Note: To help ensure that the flaxseed oil in this dressing stays fresh, since it oxidizes more quickly than other oils, break open a capsule of vitamin E, an antioxidant, and add the vitamin E oil to the dressing. Stir to combine. Be sure to store the dressing in a sealed container in the refrigerator and use within the week.

Greek Salad Dressing

Olive oil doesn't just contain healthy fats; it's also a source of potent phytonutrients that protect the arteries from injury by oxidized cholesterol.

YIELD: ABOUT ²/₃ CUP DRESSING

¹/₂ cup extra-virgin olive oil
3 tablespoons balsamic vinegar
¹/₄ teaspoon dried oregano
Salt and freshly ground black pepper

1. Put the olive oil, vinegar, and oregano in a bowl. Whisk to combine.

2. Season with salt and pepper. The touch of oregano in this vinaigrette tells you it's Greek! Enjoy on a Greek salad made with tomatoes, cucumbers, sweet peppers, black olives, and feta cheese (see page 220).

Avocado Dressing

This super-rich salad dressing is full of monounsaturated fats, the basis of the heart-healthy Mediterranean diet.

YIELD: ABOUT 1 CUP DRESSING
1 avocado
1 tablespoon minced onion
$^1/_4$ cup extra-virgin olive oil
1 tablespoon balsamic vinegar
Salt and pepper

1. Peel and pit the avocado and cut into chunks. Place the avocado chunks in a food processor fitted with a metal blade.

2. Add the onion, olive oil, and vinegar. Process until the dressing is smooth. Season with salt and pepper. Briefly process once again. Spoon this thick, rich dressing over sliced tomatoes.

What about the Wine in Wine Vinegar?

When wine is made into wine vinegar, the alcohol in the wine oxidizes and is converted into acetic acid, the component of vinegar that makes it taste sour. But this conversion is only partial and a very small amount of alcohol remains in the final wine vinegar product. If you want to be extra careful about avoiding ethanol, you can remove the last smidgeon in any wine vinegar simply by heating it. Alcohol is very volatile and evaporates in 20 to 30 seconds at 172°F, a simmering temperature.

Or perhaps you need to avoid the flavor of wine, which might trigger a relapse. Then stay away from red wine vinegar that, for instance, has a hint of cabernet or burgundy. Limit your vinegars to flavors that mask their wine origins. Rice wine vinegar is salty and sweet. Balsamic vinegar has the flavor of the oak barrel in which it's been aged.

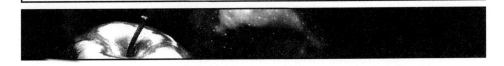

Anchovy Vinaigrette

Anchovies are an excellent source of omega-3 fatty acids, which quell inflammation, as do certain phytonutrients in olive oil.

YIELD: ABOUT 1 CUP DRESSING
2 anchovy fillets
3/4 cup extra-virgin olive oil
1/4 cup balsamic vinegar
1 teaspoon prepared mustard
Salt and pepper

1. Mince the anchovy fillets and place in a small bowl.

2. Add the olive oil, vinegar, and mustard. Season to taste with salt and pepper. Enjoy on salad greens and also use it to make potato salad. Pour the dressing on cooked potatoes while still warm, to allow the potatoes to fully absorb the flavor of the dressing.

Sesame–Yogurt Dressing

A key ingredient of this salad dressing is sesame seed paste, a staple of cooking in the Middle East, where it's called tahini. Sesame seeds are a source of B vitamins, iron, and potassium.

YIELD: ABOUT 1¹/₄ CUPS DRESSING
1/2 cup tahini
1/4 cup low-fat yogurt
2 tablespoons lemon juice
1 clove garlic, minced
1 teaspoon soy sauce
1/2 teaspoon ground cumin

1. In a small bowl, mix together the tahini, yogurt, and lemon juice.

2. Slowly add 1/2 cup of water, to thin the tahini mixture.

3. Stir in the garlic, soy sauce, and cumin. Store refrigerated.

Tomato Vinaigrette

For a quick dinner salad, start with a bag of mixed gourmet salad pieces and dress with this vinaigrette.

YIELD: ABOUT 1 CUP DRESSING
$1/4$ cup extra-virgin olive oil
1 medium-size ripe tomato, trimmed
   and quartered
3 tablespoons balsamic vinegar
2 sprigs fresh parsley, leaves only
$1/2$ teaspoon dried basil
Salt and pepper

1. Put the olive oil, tomato wedges, vinegar, parsley, and dried basil into a food processor fitted with a metal blade, or a blender.

2. Blend until the dressing is smooth, about 30 seconds. Season with salt and pepper. Refrigerate any unused dressing.

Lemon Vinaigrette

The lemon zest in this dressing contains the phytonutrient limonene, which takes part in the chemistry of the liver involved with deactivating toxins.

YIELD: ABOUT $3/4$ CUP DRESSING
1 large lemon
$1/2$ teaspoon salt
$1/2$ cup extra-virgin olive oil

1. Grate the lemon to produce 1 teaspoon of lemon zest. Halve the lemon and squeeze to yield $1/4$ cup of lemon juice. Strain the juice through a sieve to remove the seeds.

2. Mix the zest, juice, and salt in a bowl using a whisk, or in a blender or food processor. Add the oil slowly in a stream to form an emulsion. Make the dressing no more than an hour before serving, for maximum citrus flavor.

Walnut Oil Dressing

The oil in walnuts is one of the few plant sources of healing omega-3 fats and its flavor adds a tawny richness to simple salad greens. This dressing also tastes great drizzled over cooked beets.

YIELD: ABOUT 3/4 CUP DRESSING
1/2 cup walnut oil
3 tablespoons balsamic vinegar
1 teaspoon prepared mustard
Salt and pepper

1. Put the oil, vinegar, and mustard in a medium-size bowl and whisk to combine, or mix in a food processor or blender.

2. Season with salt and pepper. Make fresh for best flavor as walnut oil, because of the fragile omega-3 fats it contains, has a shorter shelf life than most oils. Refrigerate any remaining dressing in a sealed container and use within 2 or 3 days.

Desserts and Sweet Morsels

The Recipes:

Mint Chocolate–Dipped Strawberries
Baked Apples with Cranberry Chutney 🐌
Cinnamon Oranges
Poached Pears Scented with Cardamom 🐌
Apricot-Almond Crisp
Peanut Butter "Ice Cream"
Spiced Ginger Cake 🐌
Chewy Oatmeal Cookies 🐌
Broiled Spiced Dates
Fruit Salad Crepe

Eating for recovery doesn't have to stop before dessert is served. In fact, dessert is a great opportunity to eat more fruit and nuts, key foods in this nutrition program for recovery. All of the recipes that follow include one or the other, or both. Fruits such as apples and apricots contribute sweetness, and almonds and walnuts add their richness. The recipes feature these ingredients, as well as whole wheat flour, in keeping with Goal 3 of recovery eating that recommends consuming more whole foods. The only downside of these desserts is that, if you're having problems controlling blood sugar, a serving will cause a rise in blood glucose. If you find you are sugar sensitive right now in your recovery process, then just have a bite of dessert at the end of a well-balanced meal to satisfy your sweet tooth. The following recipes offer such tempting morsels as grilled dates accented with spice and chocolate-dipped strawberries.

Mint Chocolate–Dipped Strawberries

If you crave the bitter taste of coffee but are trying to cut back on how much you drink, instead have a couple of these strawberries dipped in bitter dark chocolate. Start with some that's at least 70 percent cocoa, which contains more antioxidants and feel-good chemicals than does milk chocolate. And for a gourmet treat, use a chocolate flavored with mint, such as Endangered Species brand Dark Chocolate with Deep Forest Mint, or add some fresh mint yourself, as in this recipe.

YIELD: 6 SERVINGS

3 ounces 70% dark chocolate
1 sprig fresh mint, leaves only,
    chopped finely
12 jumbo strawberries

1. Fill the bottom half of a double boiler with enough water so that the water levels falls just short of the top portion when set in the pot. Heat the water until hot and put the chocolate in the top portion of the pan. Melt the chocolate, stirring occasionally.

2. Turn off the heat beneath the double boiler. Stir the chopped mint into the chocolate.

3. Grasp a strawberry by the stem and roll it in the chocolate, coating about two-thirds of the berry. Place the dipped strawberry on a plate covered with waxed paper. Proceed with the remaining fruit.

4. Refrigerate the berries about 1 hour, or until the chocolate hardens. This sweet is best eaten the day it's prepared. Enjoy one or two as a treat at the end of a meal or as a special snack.

Baked Apples with Cranberry Chutney ㉟
(Menu 3)

Cranberries are packed with antioxidants that are good for the heart and apples give you fiber. Together, they offer good eats.

YIELD: 4 SERVINGS

4 baking apples, such as Rome, Gala, and Gravenstein

¼ cup cranberry chutney (see Note)

Preheat the oven to 350°F.

1. Core the apples almost all the way through, starting at the non-stem end.

2. Spoon chutney into the cavity of each apple.

3. Bake, uncovered, until the apples are very tender, about 1 hour. Serve warm or at room temperature.

Note: Alternate baked apple fillings include mango chutney, raisins, chopped walnuts, and pumpkin pie spice mix; or turkey or soy breakfast sausage.

Cinnamon Oranges
(Menu 17)

Sliced whole oranges are recommended for recovery over orange juice because slices, with their pith and membranes, doesn't raise blood sugar as quickly. The fiber in these slices is also good for digestion.

YIELD: 4 SERVINGS

3 navel oranges
2–3 tablespoons orange juice

¼ teaspoon ground cinnamon

1. Using a zester, cut thin strips of orange zest from half of one of the large navel oranges and set aside. Peel all the oranges and slice the fruit crosswise. Remove seeds.

2. Place the oranges in a shallow bowl. Add 2 to 3 tablespoons of orange juice and sprinkle with the cinnamon. Gently stir to distribute the spice. Let marinate for at least 1 hour, refrigerated, and serve chilled. Garnish with the orange zest.

Poached Pears Scented with Cardamom 🐚
(Menu 19)

If raw fruit seems like a chore to eat, and consequently you don't eat it, try poaching it as in this recipe, which turns an everyday pear into a succulent, gourmet delight.

YIELD: 4 SERVINGS
3 Bosc pears, ripe but not mushy
4 strips lemon zest
$1/2$ teaspoon ground cardamom

1. Peel and core the pears and cut lengthwise into $1/2$-inch-wide slices. Bring 3 cups of water to a boil in a medium-size pot and add the lemon zest, cardamom, and pears. Cover the pot and simmer until the pears are tender, at least 15 minutes. Remove the pears and place in a bowl.

2. Bring the juices in the pot to a boil and cook over medium-high heat until the sauce reduces by half. Pour through a sieve and over the pears. Serve warm, or refrigerate overnight and enjoy chilled.

Apricot–Almond Crisp
(Menu 8)

This classic comfort food dessert sends a message that you're taking good care of yourself and also gives you a serving of fruit and nuts.

YIELD: 6 SERVINGS
The topping:
$3/4$ cup almonds, chopped coarsely
$1/4$ cup whole wheat pastry flour
$1/4$ cup light brown sugar
$1/4$ teaspoon ground cinnamon
$1/8$ teaspoon grated nutmeg
$1/8$ teaspoon salt
4 tablespoons butter substitute, such as Smart Balance Buttery Spread

The fruit:
1 teaspoon cornstarch
2 teaspoon lemon juice
1 teaspoon minced lemon zest
$2^{1}/2$ pounds ripe apricots, pitted and quartered (see Note)
2 tablespoons light brown sugar
Special equipment: 8-inch square baking dish

Preheat the oven to 425°F. Grease the baking dish.

1. Put the almonds, flour, sugar, cinnamon, nutmeg, and salt in a food processor. Process until the nuts are finely chopped.

2. Melt the butter substitute in a small saucepan. Drizzle into the nut mixture and pulse a few times, until the topping resembles crumbly wet sand. Set aside.

3. Put the cornstarch, lemon juice, and lemon zest in a bowl. Mix together. Add the apricots and toss to combine. Add the sugar and toss.

4. Cover the bottom of an 8-inch square baking dish with the fruit mixture. Sprinkle the topping evenly over the apricots. Bake for 30 to 40 minutes, or until the topping is deep golden brown. Set the dish on a wire rack to cool the crisp. Serve warm.

Note: Other fruit options include apples, summer peaches, and mixed berries.

Peanut Butter "Ice Cream"

You'll be surprised how like ice cream a simple combination of bananas and peanut butter can taste, good to know about if you don't tolerate dairy foods like milk and cream. You'll need to start this dessert the day before you want to have it, to peel and then prefreeze the bananas.

YIELD: 4 SERVINGS
3 bananas, peeled and frozen
2 heaping tablespoons peanut butter
1/4 cup unsweetened applesauce

1. Slice the bananas into 1/4-inch chunks. Place in a food processor.

2. Add the peanut butter, applesauce, and 1/3 cup of water. Pulse until the bananas are cut into small bits; then process until the mixture is smooth.

3. Spoon into a bowl, cover, and place in the freezer section of a refrigerator for one hour to firm up. Serve as is or with a slice of Spiced Ginger Cake (see next recipe).

Spiced Ginger Cake 𝒱

This nourishing cake eats like a treat but also does its share in contributing to recovery, made with wholesome ingredients like whole wheat flour, sweetened with maple syrup and applesauce. And the ginger is a powerful anti-inflammatory.

YIELD: 12 SERVINGS

2 cups whole wheat pastry flour
$1/2$ cup ground almonds
$1^1/_2$ teaspoons baking soda
1 tablespoon ground ginger
1 teaspoon ground cinnamon
1 teaspoon ground allspice
$1/_4$ teaspoon grated nutmeg
$1/_4$ teaspoon salt
$1/_2$ cup raisins
$1/_2$ cup unsweetened applesauce
$1/_2$ cup 2% milk
$1/_4$ cup pure maple syrup
5 tablespoons unrefined safflower oil
Special equipment: 8-inch square
    baking dish

Preheat the oven to 350°F. Grease the baking dish.

1. Put the flour, almonds, baking soda, ginger, cinnamon, allspice, nutmeg, and salt in a bowl. Whisk together to blend. Add the raisins and mix.

2. In a second bowl, put the applesauce, milk, maple syrup, and oil. Whisk to combine.

3. Pour the wet ingredients into the flour mixture slowly and stir with a spoon. Be sure to have all the flour incorporated, but don't overmix.

4. Spoon the batter into the prepared baking dish and bake for 30 to 35 minutes. The cake is done when its top surface is springy to the touch, or a toothpick inserted into the center comes out clean. Turn out onto a wire rack to cool. Serve warm with the baked apples or poached pears, following the recipes on pages 275 and 276, or cover with plastic wrap to enjoy the next day.

Chewy Oatmeal Cookies

This is a whole-foods cookie, made without white flour or white sugar. It also gives you omega-3s in the walnuts and soluble fiber for digestive health, thanks to the oats.

YIELD: 24 COOKIES
1¹/₂ cups rolled oats
³/₄ cup whole wheat pastry flour
¹/₄ teaspoon baking powder
¹/₄ teaspoon grated nutmeg
¹/₂ teaspoon salt
1 cup chopped walnuts
¹/₂ cup Smart Balance Buttery Spread
³/₄ cup pure maple syrup
2 eggs
Special equipment: two baking
    sheets, baking parchment

Preheat the oven to 350°F. Line two baking sheets with baking parchment.

1. Put the oats, flour, baking powder, nutmeg, and salt in a large bowl. Mix together thoroughly. Add the walnuts and mix again. Set aside.

2. Put the butter substitute, maple syrup, and eggs in a food processor, and process to combine. Pour into the oat mixture. Using a spoon, mix to moisten thoroughly.

3. Drop spoonfuls of cookie dough onto the prepared baking sheets, twelve mounds per sheet.

4. Place in the preheated oven and bake for 25 minutes, until the edges of the cookies turn golden brown. Turn each cookie sheet from front to back and also switch them from top to bottom halfway through baking, to ensure even cooking.

5. Transfer the cookies, on their parchment, to cooling racks. Before peeling cookies from the parchment, let cool for at least 30 minutes.

Broiled Spiced Dates

Here's an easy way to prepare a fruit and nut combination that's sure to turn into one of your favorite snacks, with its sweet and savory flavors. Both dates and almonds supply minerals, including calcium, magnesium, and potassium. The small amount of butter in the recipe goes far, adding its special taste.

YIELD: 6 SERVINGS
12 Medjool dates
12 almonds
1 tablespoon butter, preferably
    organic
$1/4$ teaspoon ground cinnamon
$1/4$ teaspoon ground cumin
$1/8$ teaspoon salt

1. To pit the dates, slit open the top of each date, partially exposing the pit. Using your fingers, pull out the pit. Stuff each date with an almond and push the top of the date closed.

2. Melt the butter in a small saucepan. Add the cinnamon, cumin, and salt. Place the dates in the butter and turn with a spoon to coat.

3. Transfer the dates to a baking sheet and broil under heat for 10 minutes until they begin to darken. Turn once halfway through the broiling process. Savor the dates warm or at room temperature.

Fruit Salad Crepe

Ready-made crepes are a handy beginning for inventing healthy desserts made with fresh fruit. They're sold in upscale supermarkets, usually in the produce section. Use any combination of fruit to your liking, such as mangoes and pineapple or simply apples and oranges. You might also start with a bag of frozen mixed berries. Enjoy any leftover fruit salad for breakfast.

YIELD: 4 SERVINGS

2 cups fruit salad
$^1/_2$ teaspoon cornstarch
1 teaspoon Smart Balance Buttery
Spread, or more if needed

1. To prepare the fruit filling, cut the fruit salad into small bits so it can be easily folded into the crepe.

2. In a small bowl, mix together cornstarch and $^1/_4$ cup of water. Add the cut fruit and stir to combine. Put the fruit salad in a small pan and cook over medium heat for about 5 minutes, until the fruit has softened.

3. Put a small amount of butter substitute in a skillet large enough to hold the crepe. When hot, place a crepe in the pan and cook for about 7 seconds on each side, turning once with a spatula.

4. Place the warmed crepe on a dinner plate. Using $^1/_2$ cup of fruit per crepe, place a row of filling across the middle of the crepe. Using your hands, roll the crepe so that the fruit fills the crepe. Set aside and proceed with the other crepes.

5. Serve immediately as is or topped with low-fat ricotta cheese or sour cream.

Recovery Drinks

The Recipes:

Agua Fresca 🐝
Fruity Herbal Teas 🐝
Almond-Fruit Smoothie
Mango Lassi 🐝
Persian Orange Juice
Coffee-Substitute Caffe Latte
Decaf Earl Grey
Chai Spice Milk 🐝

When you're thirsty or just want to sit for a while with a cup of something, here are some beverages that fit in with the goals of recovery eating. With these drinks, you can cut back on sugar and skip the caffeine while still enjoying the experience of sipping a satisfying liquid. Drink these beverages in peaceful solitude or perhaps in the company of friends while enjoying a good conversation.

You have your choice of various sweet beverages based on fresh fruit—mixed with pure water, yogurt, and even nut butter. After you've sworn off caffeine, you can also look forward to savoring a restorative cup of black tea when you make it with a version such as decaffeinated Earl Grey. And the pleasure of a richly bitter brew that tastes almost like coffee can still be yours when you start with a product made with roasted barley and roasted chicory root. Recipes for these various beverages follow.

Plain H$_2$0

Drinking plenty of water helps in recovery by cleansing the system, brightening the mind and energizing the body, good motivations for sticking with the changes in diet now under way. Unfortunately, most people wait until they feel dry in the mouth before having a glassful, but by then the liquid is long overdue. General fatigue is an earlier sign. A good way to remind yourself to drink more water is to keep several pitchers of fresh water, along with some glasses, at strategic points around the house in easy reach and where you'll see them.

Giving yourself the purest water possible also makes good sense for recovery, sparing your liver from dealing with various toxins in the water supply. Removing chlorine and assorted pollutants and toxins makes the water more fit to drink. Invest in a top-quality water filter for your kitchen sink and take all your drinking and cooking water from this tap. Effective filters include solid carbon filters and reverse-osmosis filters.

Fruit Waters

As you become a drinker of water, of course there's nothing stopping you from having some fun with the flavor—by adding fruit. Start with a pitcher of water and add any of the following:

- ▸ Lemon slices

- ▸ Orange slices

- ▸ Lime slices

- ▸ Slices of cucumber

- ▸ A couple of strawberries

- ▸ A few chunks of watermelon

- ▸ A pineapple spear

Or go one step further and concoct what the Mexicans call an *agua fresca*, or "fresh-fruit water." This drink is made by blending ripe fruit with water. Here's the recipe:

Agua Fresca 🐏

Fruit waters are especially refreshing in hot weather as the fruit replenishes minerals lost in perspiration. This beverage also counts as at least one of your day's recommended servings of fruit.

YIELD: 4 SERVINGS

1 pound or a little more of such fruits as watermelon, peaches or pineapple, trimmed, seeds removed, and cut into chunks

2 cups filtered water
$1/2$–1 tablespoon fresh lime juice
$1/2$–1 tablespoon sugar or honey

1. Cut up about a cup's worth of the fruit into small bits to be added to the final drink later.

2. Put the remaining fruit and water into a blender and puree.

3. Using a medium-mesh strainer, strain the fruit into a pitcher with a wide opening.

4. Add lime juice and sweetener according to taste.

5. Add the chopped fruit and stir. Cover and refrigerate for at least an hour, to chill the fruit water.

6. Pour into glasses, spooning some of the chopped fruit into each. Enjoy as is or on ice.

Fruit Juice and Herbal Tea

Even though fruit juice isn't a whole food—it's missing the fruit's fiber—there are times when having a glassful hits the spot. Fruit juice is also a source of easily absorbed vitamins and minerals. Its only disadvantage is that the sugars in the juice are easily absorbed, which can cause a quick rise and then a drop in blood sugar. In someone sensitive, this can lead to mood changes and low energy. But you can easily reduce the level of sugars by mixing your fruit juice with herbal tea; with the added flavor of the tea, you won't miss the sweetness. Have fun experimenting with flavors. Try these combos and go from there.

Fruity Herbal Teas 🍵

Serve the following chilled:

- Pear juice and ginger tea

- Peach juice and mint tea

- Berry juice and hibiscus flower tea

Almond-Fruit Smoothie

The addition of almond butter to this smoothie makes it extra nourishing, adding some protein, healthy monounsaturated oils, and extra calories, and gives this fruit drink staying power, a refreshing snack that can keep you going until your next meal.

YIELD: 2 SERVINGS
2 ripe bananas, peeled and cut into
    quarters
4 fresh or frozen strawberries, stems
    removed, plus 4 for garnish
2 cups unsweetened apple juice
4 ice cubes
2 tablespoons almond butter

1. Put the bananas, strawberries, apple juice, ice cubes, and almond butter into a blender. Blend until smooth, about 15 seconds.

2. Pour the smoothie into tall, chilled glasses. Garnish each glass with a strawberry, partially split and perched on the glass rim.

Mango Lassi 🌊

Lassi is the traditional yogurt drink of India. It is served salted and savory and also sweet, made with fresh mango as in this recipe. The fruit supplies antioxidants and the yogurt aids digestion.

YIELD: 2 SERVINGS
1¹/₂ cups full-fat yogurt
1 mango, peeled and seed removed
¹/₂ teaspoon ground cumin or
   cardamom
8 ice cubes

1. Put the yogurt and mango in a blender and process for 30 seconds.

2. Add the spices and ice cubes, and continue to blend for an additional ¹/₂ minute. The yogurt should be frothy and the ice not fully disintegrated. Pour into tall glasses and serve with Indian food or as a healthful between-meal snack.

Persian Orange Juice

This is the juice version of a Middle Eastern fruit dessert—sliced oranges garnished with chopped mint and drizzled with rose water. Fresh, uncooked citrus is an excellent source of vitamin C, a fragile vitamin destroyed by heat if cooked. Mint functions as an antispasmodic, aiding digestion, and the rose water adds a touch of romance!

YIELD: 4 SERVINGS
4 cups chilled orange juice with pulp,
   not from concentrate
4 sprigs fresh mint, about 24 leaves
1 teaspoon rose water (optional) (see
   Note)

1. Put the orange juice and mint leaves into a blender. Process for about 15 seconds, until the leaves are finely chopped.

2. Stir in the rose water, adjusting the amount to taste. Pour into stemmed glasses and make a toast with this elegant drink.

Note: You'll find rose water in the spice section of some upscale markets and in Middle Eastern food shops. Rose water contains no alcohol.

Coffee-Substitute Caffe Latte

You can spare your body the strain of caffeine and still enjoy the satis-fyingly bitter flavor of coffee when you prepare a cupful with one of the new brands of coffee substitute that successfully mimics the java taste. This recipe calls for Tecchino brand, which is made with roasted chicory root, a soluble fiber whose inulin content promotes healthy mi-croflora in the gut and increases the absorption of minerals. For the complete latte effect, be sure to whirr the milk in a blender to produce some foam.

YIELD: 1 SERVING
1 teaspoon coffee substitute, such as
    Tecchino brand, or more to taste
Water for boiling
1 teaspoon sugar (optional)
3/4 cup milk
Special equipment: paper coffee filter
    and filter holder

1. Set a coffee filter holder fitted with a paper coffee filter over a coffee mug. Put the coffee substitute in the filter.

2. Boil some water and pour 1/2 cup of the boiling water through the filter and into the mug. Remove the coffee filter holder once all the water has filtered through the coffee substitute. Stir in the sugar.

3. In a small saucepan, set over medium heat, warm the milk until it begins to simmer. Pour into a blender and whip for 10 seconds to generate froth on top of the milk.

4. Pour the milk into the coffee mug, spooning froth on top of the latte. Savor immediately (see Note).

Note: For a Mexican variation on this latte, sweeten with dark brown sugar and dust the froth with ground cinnamon.

Decaf Earl Grey

You can still enjoy a tea break without giving yourself a dose of possibly jitter-making caffeine when you start with one of several decaffeinated teas on the market. This recipe gives you the time-honored technique of making a proper cup of tea with a fully developed flavor.

YIELD: 4 SERVINGS

Fresh, cold water, enough to fill a
    stove-top teakettle
5 bags decaffeinated Earl Grey
Special equipment: stove-top
    teakettle; teapot, preferably china
    rather than pottery; tea cozy
    (optional)

1. Fill the teakettle with the cold water and bring to a boil. As soon as the water boils, begin your tea making. (Boiling water for a period of time causes it to become deaerated and taste flat.)

2. Rinse the teapot with a little of the the boiling water to heat it.

3. Put the five tea bags into the teapot (one tea bag per cup you are brewing, plus one for the pot). For weaker tea, add extra hot water once the tea has brewed.

4. Pour the boiling water over the tea bags and close the pot with its lid. If you happen to have a tea cozy, also cover the entire pot with this, to hold the heat. Brew the tea for 3 minutes. When the tea has brewed, stir and pour into cups. Serve plain or with hot milk and/or sugar.

Chai Spice Milk 🍵

Indian tea, called chai, is spiked with the same spices used in Indian dishes, especially curries. Indian specialty food shops sell mixes of these spices so cooks can prepare authentic chai at home. But if you don't have a source you can easily make your own version if you have the right spices on hand. You'll need ground ginger, ground cardamom, ground cinnamon, and ground cloves. Each of these four spices also happen to have benefits for recovery: ginger is a mild stimulant and an alternative to caffeine, cardamom increases the flow of bile, cinnamon stimulates the output of gastric juices, and cloves strengthen immunity and fight infection.

YIELD: ABOUT 18 SERVINGS
2 tablespoons ground ginger
2 teaspoons ground cardamom
1 teaspoon ground cinnamon
$1/8$ teaspoon ground cloves
Milk
Water
Honey

1. Measure the spices and collect in a small jar with a lid. Close the jar and shake the spices thoroughly to mix. Store with other herbs and spices in a cool, dry place.

2. To prepare one serving, put $1/2$ teaspoon of the chai spice mixture in a mug, or use more to taste.

3. Warm the milk over medium heat in a small saucepan. Bring the water to a boil in a kettle.

4. Pour the boiling water into the mug to fill it two-thirds full. Add the warm milk and 1 teaspoon of honey. Stir and serve as an afternoon treat or at the end of an Indian meal such as the one you'll find for the Day 21 menu of the recovery diet.

7 ENHANCING RECOVERY WITH NUTRITIONAL SUPPLEMENTS

THE UNDERLYING PREMISE of this book is "food first," when it comes to repairing the physical damage caused by alcoholism. Still, nutritional supplements could have a place in the program. As you begin recovery, your body may need a boost in nutrient intake greater than diet alone can provide. Certainly, the foods recommended here can begin to make a significant difference in your nutritional status, but your recovery process may also need a jump start. As you learned in earlier chapters, alcohol abuse impairs how certain nutrients are absorbed, metabolized, and stored, and loss of liver function significantly affects nutrient status.

This chapter gives you an overview of a dozen nutritional supplements proven to be effective for recovery. Some correct nutrient deficiencies, whereas others help the system detox, reduce alcohol cravings, or do their part in restoring normal function to areas of the body damaged by alcohol abuse. Some or all of these may work for you.

The following descriptions of these supplements are designed to give you enough information about them that you can begin a conversation with your physician or a nutritionist about taking them. It is essential that you work with a health professional knowledgeable about alcohol recovery, to create a supplement regimen customized to your needs. Your physician or nutritionist will probably order lab tests to identify which vitamins and minerals are actually deficient. When ingested in high doses, nutritional supplements can have undesirable side effects. Therefore, it is not advised that you start to take these or other supplements on your own, without clearing them with a health-care professional familiar with your nutritional needs.

Minerals and Vitamins
Zinc

Both chronic and acute drinking can result in zinc deficiency. Zinc is one of the prime nutrients required for the breakdown of alcohol, which depletes the amount available for other functions, and drinking also decreases absorption of zinc while increasing urinary excretion. Foods that supply zinc may also be missing in the diet. A zinc deficiency increases the risk of developing cirrhosis of the liver and can contribute to complications of alcohol abuse, such as impaired immune function. In addition, when levels of zinc in brain tissue are low, alcoholics are more susceptible to withdrawal seizures. Supplemental zinc, coupled with vitamin C, increases alcohol detoxification. Be sure to consult with a doctor before deciding on a safe dosage.

Magnesium

It's estimated that about 60 percent of alcoholics are deficient in magnesium. Whole grains and green vegetables, excellent sources of magnesium, are probably missing in the diet and drinking increases the excretion of this mineral. Loss continues even after a person has stopped drinking and is in withdrawal. Magnesium deficiency is considered a major reason for higher risk of cardiovascular disease associated with alcoholism and low levels may also be associated with alcoholic cardiomyopathy. A German study published in 2004 in *Alcoholism: Clinical and Experimental Research* concluded that supplementing with magnesium improves sleep. During withdrawal, one of the most frequent complaints of alcoholics is sleep disturbances which can persist for months and even years. Problems with sleep are considered a predictor of relapse.

Vitamin A

Vitamin A deficiency is common in chronic alcoholics, with low levels in both the blood and the liver, where 90 percent of it is stored. Coupled with zinc deficiency, a lack of vitamin A results in ailments commonly associated with alcoholism, such as impaired immunity, skin disorders, and cirrhosis. Supplementation can result in improved night vision and sexual function, but taking vitamin A, a fat-soluble vitamin, must be done with caution. A liver damaged by alcohol is less able to store vitamin A, and vitamin A toxicity can develop. Before taking any supplement of this vitamin, consult with a physician to have your liver function assessed. If your liver is damaged, vitamin A supplementation is *not* recommended; instead eat moderate amounts of such foods as carrots and sweet potatoes, featured in the recovery menus and recipes that you'll find in chapters 5 and 6. These and many other yellow/orange foods supply beta-carotene, the water-soluble form of vitamin A that is readily excreted.

B complex

Virtually all alcoholics are deficient in at least one of the B vitamins, with at least half lacking sufficient thiamine. A severe thiamine deficiency can lead to Wernicke-Korsakoff syndrome and permanent brain damage (see chapter 2, page 25). A lack of vitamin B_6 and folic acid are also common deficiencies. Poor intake, absorption, and storage of B vitamins, as well as impaired metabolism and increased deactivation, all contribute to low levels. At the same time, drinking increases the need for these nutrients. B vitamins are available singly, or in the form of a B-complex supplement.

Antioxidants

Alcoholics are deficient in antioxidants such as vitamins C and E, and selenium. At the same time, drinking promotes the oxidation of fats and the production of destructive free radicals, increasing the need for these nutrients to prevent damage to cells. Levels of antioxidants, free radicals, and liver damage are closely related. Antioxidants also help prevent fatty infiltration of the liver.

Vitamin C. Vitamin C levels in white blood cells are directly related to the rate of clearance of alcohol in the blood. Supplementing with vitamin C speeds detoxification. In addition, taking vitamin C raises levels of glutathoine, a compound made up of amino acids that supports the liver in detoxifying pesticides and heavy metals. Glutathione helps change fat-soluble substances into water-soluble compounds so they are more easily excreted. Supplementing your diet with 500 mg of vitamin C per day maintains good tissue levels of glutathione, but taking glutathione does not.

Vitamin E. Chronic alcohol consumption leads to lower levels of vitamin E in the blood and liver. Taking a supplemental dose of this nutrient can help prevent damage to the liver and, according to a study published in 2003 in *Alcoholism: Clinical and Experimental Research*, can help prevent alcohol-related colon cancer.

Selenium. Selenium is an essential trace mineral. It works together with vitamin E to protect fat from oxidation. Selenium is safe at lower levels, but more than 900 mcg per day can be toxic.

Carnitine

Carnitine is a *liptotropic agent*, a compound that promotes the flow of fat to and from the liver. As well as facilitating the transport of fat, carnitine also promotes its breakdown. In terms of alcoholism, carnitine significantly inhibits alcohol-induced liver disease and helps prevent fatty liver. Although the body normally produces a sufficient amount of carnitine, chronic drinking interferes with this process. Alcoholism and poor diet leave the body deficient in key nutrients—vitamin C, niacin, vitamin B_6 and iron— required for carnitine production.

Glutamine

Glutamine is an amino acid that has been proven to reduce cravings for alcohol in both animal and human studies. Its ability to reduce sugar cravings has also been demonstrated. In addition, in a double-blind trial treating alcoholics, glutamine in combination with three other amino acids, phenylalanine, tyrosine, and tryptophan, plus a multivitamin-mineral supplement, lowered stress levels, as compared with the effects of a placebo, and also reduced withdrawal symptoms.

Friendly Bacteria
Probiotics

You may need to supplement your diet with beneficial strains of bacteria to reestablish healthy flora in the gut. As explained in chapter 2, alcohol abuse can lead to the colonization of the small intestine by toxin-producing bacteria. Malabsorption of such nutrients as folic acid and vitamin B_{12} can result, as well as increased intestinal permeability, which means that toxins are more easily absorbed into the system. Probiotics can prevent these problems by helping to keep toxins from entering the system. They also inhibit the reproduction of harmful bacteria, reduce the severity of gut inflammation, and lessen symptoms of lactose intolerance, all potential health issues associated with alcoholism.

Not all "healthy" bacteria are considered probiotics, only those that can survive the acidic environment of the stomach and can thrive in the intestine. The strains that are the most beneficial are L. acidophilus, bifidobacterium, and L. rhamnosus. Some probiotic supplements don't contain as much, if any, good bacteria as they claim. To maximize benefits, choose products packaged in airtight, dark brown glass bottles that are kept refrigerated in the store. You also need to refrigerate probiotics immediately once you bring them home. Their bacteria are very easily destroyed by heat.

Be sure to take probiotic supplements with meals, preferably near the end of a meal when the stomach is less acid. Then don't finish your meal with an acidic cup of coffee!

Prebiotics

Prebiotics stimulate the reproduction and activity of friendly bacteria. Fructo-oligosaccharides (FOS) are one of the most thoroughly studied prebiotics. FOS contains a mix of sugars—fructose and glucose—that ferment and stimulate the growth of bifidobacteria in the colon. While no optimal dose has been identified, FOS is well tolerated in doses up to 10 grams per day; however, taken in excess, it causes stomach cramps and bloating. (For more on FOS, see chapter 3, page 51.)

Herbs
Silymarin

Silymarin is a respected herbal treatment for alcohol-related liver disease, ranging from mild to serious cirrhosis. It is the active compound in milk thistle, a plant commonly found growing wild, and has been used medicinally for over two thousand years. It consists of a complex of flavonoids, water-soluble plant pigments, and is extracted from the dried fruit of the plant. Silymarin is a powerful antioxidant and blocks development of cirrhosis. In double-blind studies, it's been demonstrated that silymarin regenerates injured liver cells once a person stops drinking. And in other research, for patients with liver disease, supplementing with silymarin extended life span.

Silymarin is virtually free of side effects, even for pregnant and breast-feeding women, and can be used long term to treat chronic liver disease. Positive results can be expected beginning in eight to twelve weeks. Select a supplement based on an extract of milk thistle standardized to 80 percent silymarin content.

Remember, if you do start taking any of these supplements or others, they are just that, *supplements*—they don't replace food. You still need enough of the three major nutrients—carbohydrates, protein, and fat—to survive and recover; that is, you need to eat! This book supplies you with a ready-made means of restoring your health with food, as you follow the selection suggestions and try the recipes. You can take a powerful step toward recovery as soon as your next meal!

ACKNOWLEDGMENTS

M ANY HEARTFELT THANKS to everyone at Da Capo Press and the team that helped bring this book to light: Renee Sedliar, senior editor, who generously and kindly helped shape the book, asked the right questions, and assisted me with the answers; Iris Bass, who copyedited the text, adding important points and fine-tuning for clarity; Cisca L. Schreefel, senior project editor, who kept the production process on track; Wendie Carr, expert publicist, who spread the word; and Matthew Lore, vice president and executive editor, who saw the possibilities of the subject and agreed to publication. Thank you, too, to the home team—the many dear friends who cheered for me as I wrote, and my husband, Victor Watson, who supported me in every way.

HEALTHY FOOD RESOURCES

WHILE I CAN'T TAKE you with me to the market, I can give you this list of some of the most delicious and healthy food products out there for you to explore.

Meat, Poultry, and Meat Substitutes

EBERLY POULTRY FARMS

www.eberlypoultry.com

free-range poultry, fed organic grains, antibiotic and growth stimulant free, raised on GMO-free feed and pure water

Eberly offers a complete line of organic and natural poultry products, including hard-to-find specialty items such as geese, Mallard ducks, partridge, rabbit, and quail, as well as smoked whole turkeys and smoked chicken breasts.

APPLEGATE FARMS

www.applegatefarms.com

organic hot dogs—chicken, beef, or turkey

Applegate's products are uncured, and antibiotic and nitrite-free.

MESQUITE FOODS

www.mesquiteorganicbeef.com

certified-organic grass-fed beef

This beef is low in saturated fat and high in omega-3 fatty acids compared with conventionally raised beef, and is not raised with hormones or antibiotics.

PANORAMA GRASS-FED MEATS

www.panoramameats.com

grass-fed beef, raised without hormones or antibiotics

Compared with grain-fed beef, Panorama contains 60 percent more omega-3s, twice as much vitamins A and E, and a higher concentration of unsaturated fats versus saturated fats.

ORGANIC PRAIRIE FAMILY OF FARMS

www.organicprairie.com

fresh beef, ham, turkey, and hot dogs; premium choice beef and heirloom pork; frozen beef steak and patties, liver, hot dogs, pork chops, pork links, ham, Italian pork sausage, whole and ground chicken and turkey, boneless chicken breasts, chicken hot dogs

The farm's organic meat and poultry products are from animals raised without antibiotics and synthetic hormones.

SHELTON'S

www.sheltons.com

free-range chickens and turkeys

Shelton's poultry is free of antibiotics, hormones, and artificial growth stimulants and processed by hand.

SOMMERS ORGANIC

www.sommersorganic.com

unique line of frozen meat products, including organic pork chops, rib-eye steak, and burgers as well as fully cooked meats, such as seasoned pot roast and prime rib

Grown and raised without hormones, antibiotics, or chemical additives, each cooked product is wrapped for quick and easy preparation.

BOCA

www.bocaburger.com

veggie burgers and more: meatless breakfast wraps with soy protein, egg white, and cheese; breakfast links and patties; lasagna; and Hot & Spicy Chik'n Wings

Boca uses no artificial preservatives or flavors.

Seafood

HENRY & LISA'S

www.henryandlisas.com

canned wild Alaskan pink salmon and solid white albacore tuna, both cooked only once in natural oils for higher omega-3 content; organic white shrimp; Celebrity Chef Entrées: Wild Salmon with Asian Ginger Marinade, Bay Scallops with Japanese Glaze, Wild South American Mahimahi with Caribbean Marinade

Henry & Lisa's sells premium-grade natural fish, caught and cultured by artisanal fishers, from well-managed wild fisheries and responsible aquaculture.

OMEGA FOODS LTD.

www.omegafoods.net

frozen, wild-caught salmon burgers, tuna burgers, mahimahi burgers, shrimp burgers, hors d'oeuvre–size Tomato Basil Salmon Bites

Omega's chopped fillets are high in protein and low in carbs, and contain no dairy, wheat, or preservatives.

First-Class Treats

CHOCTÁL, INC.

www.Choctal.com

Chocolate ice cream made with named-origin cocoa powders, such as organic Dominican cocoa, as well as exceptionally delicious Madagascar Vanilla ice cream

If you are going to indulge in a rich dessert, have the best.

ENDANGERED SPECIES

www.chocolatebar.com

chocolate bars available in 39 percent to a whopping 88 percent cocoa

The higher the percent of cocoa, the more phytonutrients the candy contains; 10 percent of net profits are donated to help support species, habitat, and humanity.

Frozen Entrées

CEDARLANE NATURAL FOODS

www.cedarlanefoods.com

an extensive line of international dishes such as Mexican tamales and Greek moussaka as well as various dinner entrées, focaccia, burritos, appetizers, and snacks

Cedarlane's products are all natural and vegetarian, and many are made with organic ingredients.

TANDOOR CHEF

a complete line of Indian dishes, both vegetarian and nonvegetarian, as well as bread and appetizers

Tandoor Chef provides a quick meal at home that tastes like you're eating out; you'll benefit from the variety of healthful ingredients that Indian cuisine offers.

AMY'S KITCHEN

www.amys.com

an extensive range of vegetarian dishes from pizzas and veggie burgers to pot pies and toaster pop-ups; Asian, Mexican, and Indian dishes; and whole meals

These products are made with natural and organic ingredients; nongluten and dairy-free items are also available.

MOOSEWOOD

www.fairfieldfarmkitchens.com

frozen vegetarian entrées: Chilaquile Casserole (cheese, tomatoes, and red beans), Macaroni & Three Cheeses, Moroccan Stew, plus refrigerated soups

Moosewood uses organic local and regional ingredients; the entrées come in microwavable heat-and-serve containers.

Side Dishes and Special Ingredients

EARTHLY DELIGHTS

www.earthlydelightsorganics.com

organic jarred fruits, including pineapple chunks, papaya chunks, and fruit cocktail

Premium hand-selected fruit is hand-picked, hand-cut, and packed with care in its own natural juices with no added sugar.

CASCADIAN FARM

www.cascadianfarm.com

full line of organic frozen fruit and vegetables (both single and combinations), plus new vegetable products designed to be heated by steaming, as well as fruit spreads, pickles, and granola bars
Several vegetable combos come with gourmet flavorings.

SNOPAC

www.snopac.com

frozen organic vegetables and fruit, including cut spinach, mixed vegetables, blueberries, whole cranberries, Southern-Style Hashbrowns, and Soycutash made with soybeans, corn, and red peppers
SnoPac's produce is organically grown and processed, harvested at the right time for top flavor.

MUIR GLEN

www.muirglen.com

canned tomatoes, sauces, and soups such as chicken and wild rice
Thanks to organic ingredients, flavor of Muir Glen's canned tomatoes is superior to most fresh tomatoes; these products are a must for the kitchen pantry.

FRANNY'S

www.frannysorganic.com
huge, sumptuous raisins made from red and green seedless grapes
Franny's jumbo raisins are organic and specially dried to make them extra plump and juicy.

Beverages

TROPICANA

www.tropicana.com
organic orange juice and organic Orchard Medley made with apples and pears
Beverages are made with 100 percent pure and natural juices.

CERES

www.ceresjuices.com

all-natural exotic juices, including peach, pear, mango, and litchi

Packed in aseptic cartons, these 100-percent juice beverages are produced in the Ceres Valley near Cape Town in South Africa and have no added sugar or preservatives.

SONOMA SPARKLER

www.sonomacider.com

nonalcoholic sparkling juices, including sparkling apple-raspberry, pear and blood orange, plus organic apple sparkler and organic lemonade sparkler

These products are processed in small batches, apple based, and 100 percent juice.

APPLE & EVE

www.appleandeve.com

juice and juice blends, including vintage Concord, cranberry-blueberry, lemonade–green tea, and pomegranate

Apple & Eve sells 100 percent pure organic juice.

L & A

www.langers.com

100 percent juice, including papaya-pineapple, pineapple-coconut, and hibiscus cooler

L & A's juices have no added sugar, preservatives, or artificial ingredients.

AMY & BRIAN

info@marketconnectionsgroup.com

all-natural isotonic coconut juice

This "water"' from young coconuts is unsweetened and naturally high in potassium and magnesium, excellent for electrolyte replacement.

NUMI

www.numitea.com

hand-blended organic full-leaf teas, including aged Earl Grey, decaffeinated black tea, white teas, and caffeine-free herbal teasans, such as Moroccan mint and spiced rooibos

Numi's teas have no added oils or flavorings, and come in GMO biodegradable tea bags.

Dairy

MOUNTAIN HIGH

www.mountainhighyogurt.com

all-natural yogurt with no artificial sweeteners, flavors, colors, starches, or preservatives

Mountain High's yogurts contain billions of live, active, and probiotic cultures—a unique blend of L. acidophilus, B. bifidus, and L. casei.

CASCADE FRESH

www.cascadefresh.com

sour cream, Greek- and Mediterranean-style yogurts, fruit smoothies

Made in small batches and growth hormone, preservative, and antibiotic free, Cascade Fresh's yogurts include eight active probiotic cultures; their smoothies contain no refined sugar.

Snacks

SEAPOINT FARMS

www.seapointfarms.com

dry-roasted edamame (soybeans), spicy or lightly salted

Seapoint's edamame is high in protein and isoflavones, and low in carbs and fat, as well as non-GMO.

LUNDBERG

www.lundberg.com

whole-grain brown rice chips in many flavors, including wasabi and Santa Fe barbecue

Lundberg's rice chips are all natural and part of a large line of quality rice products worth exploring.

Oils

MIDDLE EARTH ORGANICS

100 percent organic, cold-pressed extra-virgin olive oil

Middle Earth's oils have a high antioxidant content and extra-smooth flavor, and are packaged in dark, corked bottles to prevent deterioration by light and air.

UDO'S CHOICE

www.florahealth.com

3-6-9 oil blend that supplies a balance of heart-healthy oils

Udo's oil is a source of omega-9s derived from algae rather than fish.

Sweeteners and Flavorings

STEVITA CO.

www.stevitastevia.com

a range of stevia products, including spoonable and liquid forms

Stevia is an herb up to three hundred times sweeter than sugar, yet with a negligible effect on blood sugar.

ORGANIC BLUE AGAVE

www.OrganicSyrups.biz

nectar of the blue agave, a cactuslike plant native to Mexico, with a rich, full taste

Agave is 25 percent sweeter than regular sugar but has a low glycemic index.

COOK'S VANILLA POWDER

www.cooksvanilla.com

vanilla bean extractives in a dextrose base

The benefit of this vanilla product for recovery is that it is alcohol-free.

RECOMMENDED READING

Glycemic Index and Glycemic Load Reference Books

Brand-Miller, J., W., M. S. Thomas, K. Foster-Powell, and S. Colagiuri. *The New Glucose Revolution*. New York: Marlowe & Company, 2007.

Thompson, Rob. *The Glycemic Load Diet*. New York: McGraw-Hill, 2006.

Cookbooks

Bittman, Mark. *How to Cook Everything*. New York: Macmillan, 1998.

Editors of *Cook's Illustrated*. *The Best Recipe*. Brookline: Boston Common Press, 1999.

Hensperger, Beth. *Not Your Mother's Slow Cooker Recipes for Two*. Boston: Harvard Common Press, 2007.

Jaffrey, Madhur, and Noel Barnhurst. *Madhur Jaffrey's Quick and Easy Indian Cooking*. San Francisco: Chronicle Books, 2007.

Siple, Molly. *Healing Foods for Dummies*. Foster City: IDG Books Worldwide, 1999.

ORGANIZATIONS FOR ALCOHOLISM AND RECOVERY

ADDICTION INSTITUTE OF NEW YORK

1000 Tenth Avenue
New York, NY 10019
212-523-6491
www.AddictionInstituteNY.org

ADULT CHILDREN OF ALCOHOLICS

P.O. Box 3216
Torrance, CA 90510
310-534-1815
www.adultchildren.org

AL-ANON/ALATEEN FAMILY GROUPS

1600 Corporate Landing Parkway
Virginia Beach, VA 23454
1-888-4AL-ANON
1-757-563-1600
www.al-anon.alateen.org or www.Al-AnonFamilyGroups.org

ALCOHOLICS ANONYMOUS (AA)

475 Riverside Drive
New York, NY 10115
212-870-3400
www.aa.org

THE BETTY FORD CENTER

39000 Bob Hope Drive
Rancho Mirage, CA 92270
760-773-4100
800-434-7365
www.bettyfordcenter.org

JOIN TOGETHER

715 Albany Street, 580–3rd Floor
Boston, MA 02118
617-437-1500
www.jointogether.org

NATIONAL ASSOCIATION FOR CHILDREN OF ALCOHOLICS

11426 Rockville Pike, Suite 100
Rockville, MD 20852
301-468-0985
www.nacoa.org

NATIONAL CLEARINGHOUSE FOR ALCOHOL AND DRUG INFORMATION

P.O. Box 2345
Rockville, MD 20847–2345
1-800-729-6686
http://ncadi.samhsa.gov

NATIONAL COUNCIL ON ALCOHOLISM AND DRUG DEPENDENCE, INC. (NCADD)

12 West 21st Street, 7th floor
New York, NY 10017
800-NCA-CALL
800-622-2255
www.ncadd.org

NATIONAL INSTITUTE ON ALCOHOL ABUSE AND ALCOHOLISM

5635 Fishers Lane, MSC 9304

Bethesda, MD 20892–9304

301-443-3860

www.niaaa.nih.gov

THE PARTNERSHIP FOR A DRUG-FREE AMERICA

405 Lexington Avenue, Suite 1601

New York, NY 10174

212-922-1560

www.drugfree.org

SELECTED BIBLIOGRAPHY

Barak, A. J., H. C. Beckenhauer, and D. J. Tuma. "Betaine, Ethanol, and the Liver: A Review." *Alcohol* 13, no. 4 (1996): 395–98.

Beckman, L. J., and K. T. Ackerman. "Women, Alcohol and Sexuality." *Recent Developments in Alcohol* 12 (1995): 267–85.

Bennett, J. W. "The Interpretation of Pueblo Culture." *Southwestern Journal of Anthropology* 2, no. 3 (1946): 361–74.

Biery, J. R., J. H. Williford, and E. A. McMullen. "Alcohol Craving in Rehabilitation: Assessment of Nutritional Therapy." *Journal of the American Dietetic Association* 91 (1991): 463–66.

Blasco, C., et al. "Prevalence and Mechanisms of Hyperhomocysteinemia in Chronic Alcoholics." *Alcoholism: Clinical and Experimental Research* 29, no. 6 (2005): 1044–48.

Blumenthal, Roger S., and Simeon Margolis. The Johns Hopkins White Papers, Heart Attack Prevention, 2006.

Bode, C., and J. C. Bode. "Alcohol's Role in Gastrointestinal Tract Disorders." *Alcohol Health & Research World* 21, no. 1 (1997): 76–83.

_____. "Effect of Alcohol Consumption on the Gut." *Best Practice & Research: Clinical Gastroenterology* 17, no. 4 (2003): 575–92.

Breslow, R. A., Patricia M. Guenther, and B. A. Smothers. "Alcohol Drinking Patterns and Diet Quality: The 1999–2000 National Health and Nutrition Examination Survey." *American Journal of Epidemiology* 163, no. 4 (2006): 359–66.

Brostoff, Jonathan, and Linda Gamlin. *The Complete Guide to Food Allergy and Intolerance.* New York: Crown Publishers, 1989.

Bubout, D. "Nutritional and Metabolic Effects of Alcoholism: Their Relationship with Alcoholic Liver Disease." *Nutrition* 15, nos. 7–8 (1999): 583–89.

Butterworth, R. F. "Hepatic Encephalopathy." *Alcohol Research and Health* 27, no. 3 (2003): 240–46.

Bujanda, I. "The Effects of Alcohol Consumption upon the Gastrointestinal Tract." *American Journal of Gastroenterology* 95, no. 12 (2000): 3374–82.

Callaci, J. J., et al. "The Effects of Binge Alcohol Exposure on Bone Resorption and Biomechanical and Structural Properties Are Offset by Concurrent Bisphosphonate Treatment." *Alcoholism: Clinical and Experimental Research* 28, no. 1 (2004): 182–91.

Crews, F. T., et al. "Alcohol-Induced Neurodegeneration: When, Where and Why?" *Alcoholism: Clinical and Experimental Research* 28, no. 2 (2004): 350–64.

Editorial. *New England Journal of Medicine* 320, no. 7 (1989): 458–59.

Foster-Powell, K., S. H. Holt, and J. C. Brand-Miller. "International Table of Glycemic Index and Glycemic Load Values: 2002." *American Journal of Clinical Nutrition* 76, no. 1 (2002): 5–56.

Gaby, Alan R., and the Healthnotes medical team. *The Natural Pharmacy.* New York: Three Rivers Press, 2006.

Gavaler, J. S. "Alcohol and Nutrition in Postmenopausal Women." *Journal of the American College of Nutrition* 12, no. 4 (1993): 349–56.

Gonzalez-Reimers, E., et al. "Rib Fractures in Chronic Alcoholic Men: Relationship with Feeding Habits, Social Problems, Malnutrition, Bone Alterations, and Liver Dysfunction." *Alcohol* 37, no. 2 (2005): 113–17.

Guenther, R. M. "Role of Nutritional Therapy in Alcoholism Treatment." *International Journal for Biosocial Research* 4 (1983): 5–18.

Gunzerath, L., et al. "National Institute on Alcohol Abuse and Alcoholism Report on Moderate Drinking." *Alcoholism: Clinical and Experimental Research* 28, no. 6 (2004): 829–47.

Halsted, C. H., A. E. Robles, and E. Mezey. "Distribution of Ethanol in the Human Gastrointestinal Tract." *American Journal of Clinical Nutrition* 26 (1973): 831–34.

Hernandez-Avila, M., et al. Caffeine, "Moderate Alcohol Intake, and Risk of Fractures of the Hip and Forearm in Middle-aged Women." *American Journal of Clinical Nutrition* 54 (1991): 157–63.

Lark, Susan M., and James A. Richards. *The Chemistry of Success.* San Francisco: Bay Books, 2000.

Larmarche, F., et al. "Influence of Vitamin E, Sodium Selenite, and Astrocyte-Conditioned Medium on Neuronal Survival after Chronic Exposure to Ethanol." *Alcohol* 33 (2004): 127–38.

Larson, Joan Mathews. *Seven Weeks to Sobriety.* New York: Random House, 1997.

Lieber, C. S. "Alcohol, Liver, and Nutrition." *Journal of the American College of Nutrition* 10, no. 6 (1991): 602–32.

_____. Herman Award Lecture, 1993: "A Personal Perspective on Alcohol, Nutrition and the Liver." *American Journal of Clinical Nutrition* 58 (1993): 430–42.

_____. "Alcohol: Its Metabolism and Interaction with Nutrients." *Annual Review of Nutrition* 20 (2000): 395–430.

Mann, R. E., Reginald G. Smart, and R. Govoni. "The Epidemiology of Alcoholic Liver Disease." *Alcohol Research and Health* 27, no. 3 (2003): 209–19.

Marlett, Judith A. "Content and Composition of Dietary Fiber in 117 Frequently Consumed Foods." *Journal of the American Dietetic Association* 92 (1992): 175–86.

Martin, P. R., C. K. Singleton, and S. Hiller-Sturmhöfel. "The Role of Thiamine Deficiency in Alcohol Brain Disease." *Alcohol Research & Health* 27, no. 2 (2003): 134–42.

Mathews-Larsen, J., and R. A. Parker. "Alcoholism Treatment with Biochemical Restoration as a Major Component." *International Journal for Biosocial Research* 9, no. 1 (1987): 92–106.

Minugh, A. P., C. Rice, and L. Young. "Gender, Health Beliefs, Health Behaviors, and Alcohol Consumption." *American Journal of Drug and Alcohol Abuse* 24, no. 3 (1998): 483–98.

Neuman, Manuela G. "Cytokines—Central Factors in Alcoholic Liver Disease." *Alcohol Research & Health* 27, no. 4 (2003): 307–16.

Nijhoff, W. A., et al. "Effects of Consumption of Brussels Sprouts on Intestinal and Lymphocytic Glutathione S-Transferases in Humans." *Carcinogenesis* 16, no. 9 (1995): 2125–28.

Oscar-Berman, M., and K. Marinkovic. "Alcoholism and the Brain: An Overview." *Alcohol Research & Health* 27, no. 2 (2003): 125–33.

Pawlosky, R. J., and S. Salem, Jr. "Alcohol Consumption in Rhesus Monkeys Depletes Tissues of Polyunsaturated Fatty Acids and Alters Essential Fatty Acid Metabolism." *Alcoholism: Clinical and Experimental Research* 23, no. 2 (1999): 311–17.

Petri, A. L., et al. "Alcohol Intake, Type of Beverage, and Risk of Breast Cancer in Pre-and Postmenopausal Women." *Alcoholism: Clinical and Experimental Research* 28, no. 7 (2004): 1084–90.

Pizzorno, Joseph, and Michael T. Murray. *Encyclopedia of Natural Medicine*. New York: Three Rivers Press, 1998.

Preedy, V. R., T. J. Peters, and H. Shy. "Metabolic Consequences of Alcohol Dependency." *Adverse Drug Reaction Toxicology Review* 16, no. 4 (1997): 235–56.

Preedy, V. R., et al. "Protein Metabolism in Alcoholism: Effects on Specific Tissues and the Whole Body." *Nutrition* 15, nos. 7–8 (July–August 1999): 604–8.

Randolph, Theron G., and Ralph W. Moss. *An Alternative Approach to Allergies*. New York: Harper & Row, 1989.

Reynolds, K., et al. "Alcohol Consumption and Risk of Stroke." *Journal of the American Medical Association* 289, no. 5 (2003): 579–88.

Ridker, Paul M., et al. "C-Reactive Protein and Other Markers of Inflammation in the Prediction of Cardiovascular Disease in Women." *New England Journal of Medicine* 342, no. 12 (2000): 836–43.

Rivlin, S. Richard. "Magnesium Deficiency and Alcohol Intake: Mechanisms, Clinical Significance and Possible Relation to Cancer Development (A Review)." *Journal of the American College of Nutrition* 13, no. 5 (1994): 416–23.

Salem, N. Jr., et al. "Mechanisms of Action of Docosahexaenoic Acid in the Nervous System." *Lipids* 36, no. 9 (2001): 945–59.

Schenker, S. and M. K. Bay. "Alcohol and Endotoxin: Another Path to Alcohol Liver Injury?" *Alcoholism: Clinical and Experimental Research* 19, no. 5 (1995): 1364–66.

Scribner, K. B., D. B. Pawlak, and D. S. Ludwig. "Hepatic Steatosis and Increased Adiposity in Mice Consuming Rapidly vs. Slowly Absorbed Carbohydrate." *Obesity* 15, no. 9 (2007): 2190–99.

Syapin, Peter J., William F. Hickey, and Cynthia J. M. Kane. "Alcohol Brain Damage and Neuroinflammation: Is There a Connection?" *Alcoholism: Clinical and Experimental Research* 29, no. 6 (2005): 1080–89.

Taniguchi, N., and S. Kaneko. "Alcoholic Effect on Male Sexual Function." *Nippon Rinsho* 55, no. 11 (1997): 3040–44.

Tenth Special Report to the U.S. Congress on Alcohol and Health, U.S. Department of Health and Human Services, Public Health Service, National Institutes of Health, National Institute on Alcohol Abuse and Alcoholism, June 2000.

Thompson, Warren G. "Coffee: Brew or Bane?" *American Journal of the Medical Sciences* 308, no. 1 (1994): 49–57.

Turner, R. T. "Skeletal Response to Alcohol." *Alcoholism: Clinical and Experimental Research* 24, no. 11 (2000): 1693–1701.

Werbach, M. R. "Alcohol Craving." *International Journal of Alternative and Complementary Medicine* (July 1993): 32.

_____. *Nutritional Influences on Illness*. Tarzana, CA: Third Line Press, 1993.

Wu, D., and A. I. Cederbaum. "Alcohol, Oxidative Stress, and Free Radical Damage." *Alcohol Research & Health* 27, no. 4 (2003): 277–84.

Yoshitsugu, M., and M. Ihori. "Endocrine Disturbances in Liver Cirrhosis—Focused on Sex Hormones." *Nippon Rinsho* 55, no. 11 (1997): 3002–6.

Zhang, X. "Ethanol and Acetaldyhyde in Alcoholic Cardiomyopathy: From Bad to Ugly en Route to Oxidative Stress." *Alcohol* 32 (2004): 175–86.

INDEX

P-age numbers in italics refer to information in text boxes.